# Big Fit Girl

# Big Fit Girl

FOREWORD BY
**Jess Weiner**

Embrace the
Body You Have

## LOUISE GREEN

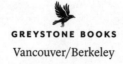

**GREYSTONE BOOKS**

Vancouver/Berkeley

Greystone Books Ltd.
www.greystonebooks.com

Cataloguing data available from Library and Archives Canada
ISBN 978-1-77164-212-5 (pbk.)
ISBN 978-1-77164-213-2 (epub)

Editing by Nancy Flight
Copyediting by Jennifer Croll
Proofreading by Jennifer Stewart
Cover design by Peter Cocking
Text design by Nayeli Jimenez
Cover photograph by Vairdy Photography
Printed and bound in Canada on ancient-forest-friendly paper by Friesens

We gratefully acknowledge the support of the Canada Council for the
Arts, the British Columbia Arts Council, the Province of British Columbia
through the Book Publishing Tax Credit, and the Government of Canada
for our publishing activities.

Canadä

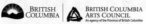

Canada Council   Conseil des arts
for the Arts     du Canada

The advice in this book has been carefully considered and checked by the
author and publisher. It should not, however, be regarded as a substitute
for medical advice. We recommend talking to your doctor before starting
any new exercise routine.

*For Chris for showing me what is possible and for all the big girls who are ready to live their athletic dreams. I believe in you.*

# CONTENTS

# FOREWORD

FOR THE PAST two decades, I've focused my personal and professional energy on the betterment of women and girls, helping them find their own road to self-discovery and confidence. Much like a personal trainer for the mind, I've developed curriculums and exercises, clocking countless miles working alongside teens, moms, and everyday women around the world, showing them how to flex their self-esteem muscles, adopt a healthy mindset, and nurture a strong self-image. Admittedly, even my own path has navigated bumps and sharp turns. While I've always considered myself athletic, my body type didn't necessarily fit the mold of what our culture would consider an "athletic build."

Reflecting back on the decades of my life, fitness served me in different ways, which in turn directly impacted how I felt in my body. I've now realized that my body wasn't just a vessel that helped me reach my fitness goals—it served as a catalyst for change. Good change. Necessary change. Regardless of my age, I've learned to never let the size of my body stop me from moving it.

In my twenties, I challenged preconceived notions of what my body could endure. At age twenty-six and a size 16, I ran my first marathon. I didn't do it to place, I did it to finish and to accomplish a goal that I never thought possible while raising funds and awareness for an AIDS charity I was involved with. As I closed in on the finish line nearly eight hours into the race, the large crowds that once served as my motivation had dissipated, and my body was crippled with fatigue. I pushed myself to cross the line and looking back, I now realize how I worked *with* my body to achieve my goal. We were partners; my body didn't have to be my enemy after all.

As I moved into my thirties, I found fitness to be a curative escape from what was happening in my life After a very long relationship that culminated in a dramatic breakup, I was single and needed something to balance the rollercoaster of emotions I was facing. Call it rebound therapy, but I decided to take on pole dancing. It was a liberating exercise and allowed me to find a sensual softness I had lost during the long-term relationship. Yet again, my body proved it could do things I never thought possible.

Today, at forty-two, I look at health and my relationship with my body in a different way. My focus is less on my body's appearance and more on its longevity. I'm married to the love of my life and together, we choose to see fitness as a way to express our care for ourselves and each other.

I treat the entire concept of moving my body differently now. Essentially, I look for ways to motivate myself to care for my body to allow me to prolong living this incredible life I've created. The answer for me lately has been boxing. It not only serves as a physical workout, but also a way for me to mentally train, de-stress, and pound out over two decades of negative thoughts. When I lace up the gloves, I'm looking to build power, stamina, and mental fortitude more so than trying to improve muscle definition. Regardless, boxing is a never-ending fitness challenge that allows me to push my limits.

No matter what road you've traveled in your relationship with your body and wellness, I believe in an infinite number of "do-overs." It is always the right time to redefine your connection to moving, growing, and developing a deep self-appreciation for everything your body (whatever its appearance) allows you to do.

In this love letter to our inner athletes, Louise inspires us to challenge labels and cultural perceptions. From sharing her own personal journey to providing step-by-step guidance on how to build both our mental and physical stamina, *Big Fit Girl* shows us how to work *with*, not against our bodies—regardless of shape and size. She reminds us that the "why" is just as important as the "how" when it comes to exercise. Read along as Louise shows us how to defy stereotypes, embrace our bodies, and squash our own limitations.

Your body, heart, and mind will thank you for it.

Yours in empowerment,
JESS WEINER

# Finding My Way to Limitless

IN MY EARLY twenties, this was my life: I drank alcohol excessively, smoked cigarettes, and regularly ate greasy Chinese food from the mall food court. I was mostly sedentary: I worked a desk job, and my evenings revolved around my couch and several glasses of wine. The only time I exercised was in fleeting three-day bursts in an attempt to fix my unhealthy lifestyle.

No matter how hard I tried to change, I would fall off the wagon and revert to my old habits. I promised myself every single night that the next day would be different. It never was. What was I doing wrong? My sporadic and extreme attempts to incorporate fitness and healthy eating into my life were accompanied by a heavy dose of self-loathing, and I became trapped in a vicious cycle of indulgence and self-denial.

Most days I woke up hung over. As I pulled myself out of bed, my body felt like it weighed a thousand pounds. I would take a long shower to try to wash it all away—the nicotine that lingered on my skin, the feelings of self-hatred, the fatigue.

Standing in front of the mirror, I would ask myself: "How did I get here?"

I felt a great deal of anxiety due to my lack of self-control and the impact my unhealthy habits had on my body. I felt trapped and unfulfilled, a long way from the "ideal" woman I imagined I could be. During my days working a job I didn't love, I projected the image of a happy, normal young woman. I would push down my internal upheaval and put on a smile. I hung out with friends, attended office functions, and spent time with my boyfriend. On the outside, things looked fairly normal. On the inside, I was full of sadness and turmoil.

At the time, I worked at a downtown law firm. Each morning on my way to work I walked past high-end fashion stores, windows glistening with shiny, large-scale posters of long, lean supermodels. Athletic apparel stores displayed photos of tanned, toned women wearing nearly nothing over their perfect skin. The women in these pictures seemed to have it together. I did not.

I lived this way for nearly a decade. I consumed junk food, alcohol, and cigarettes to smother my bad feelings. This only made me more resentful and self-blaming because I could never reach my ideal self. My life was limited in every way. I thought the way out was to lose weight and shape myself into the feminine ideal that bombarded me from every direction: if only I too could be a size 4, happiness would shine down on me.

I tried counting calories, fat grams, and points. I avoided carbs, ate nothing but cabbage soup, survived on protein shakes, and consumed only pre-packaged diet foods. I restricted my food intake and then binged from white-knuckled deprivation. None of it worked. It only made me feel worse.

I felt alone, broken, and full of shame. I didn't yet know that I was one among countless women in this spin cycle of diet routines. Maybe you can relate. Maybe that is why you picked up this book.

In 2012, a report by ABC News revealed that 108 million Americans were actively dieting at the time.[1] These dieters, roughly a third of the U.S. population, 85 percent of whom are women, will make four to five attempts each year to lose weight. These women are real people, just like you and me. They have hopes and dreams. They feel stuck, just like I did, and perhaps just like you do now.

Dieting will likely never be the thing that makes us happy and free.

To triumph, we need to resolve what might be broken inside us and shine a light on what drives us to believe that our value depends on our dress size. It all comes back to our cultural perceptions of weight. The diet industry reaps approximately 20 billion dollars off the weight-loss efforts of dieters. Statistics show that only 5 percent of dieters will make it to their ideal weight and maintain it for five or more years. The diet industry's profit model depends on the failure of people like you and me.

Why do we continue to buy in? Why did I starve myself, binge from deprivation, and succumb to every gimmick on the market? I was desperate to fit in. Perhaps you feel this way too. We live in a culture obsessed with a feminine ideal that is extremely thin. I don't blame you. I don't blame me. This is not our fault. Our society imposes these beliefs on us and at the root of all our insecurities is the weight-loss industry's money-making machine.

I FANTASIZED ABOUT being the slim, athletic woman in the fitness store windows. I signed on the dotted line for a gym membership many times. I paid the fee every month but found gym culture intimidating and never went. Sometimes I went so far as to drive to the track before work. I smoked on the way over, trying to stifle the negative chatter in my head. I would attempt to run a few laps, breathing heavily and exhaling boozy breath, only to call it a day and light another cigarette. In those moments I remembered my athletic childhood, and as I smoked while the sun rose, I wondered what had happened to me.

Change came only when I hit rock bottom. Maybe you feel like you are there right now. It is a desperate and lonely place to be, but it is a position from which the only direction is up. From rock bottom, you can rise and build something new. At the age of twenty-nine, I made a conscious decision to change my life: to throw out the habits that were preventing me from being healthy and happy. I decided to adopt new, positive habits.

I had always dreamed of being a runner, even though I had never witnessed a woman like me achieving athletic feats. I found a local running program and resolved to reach for my athletic dreams, no matter what it took. This was the first step. Though I didn't have a role model for an athlete in a bigger body I was determined to find her—or to create her. I didn't have to wait long; I only had to look in the right place.

I signed up for a "Learn to Run 5K" group offered by my local running store. My desire to change my life had become stronger than my desire to stay in my comfort zone, and a new identity was brewing. There was a reckless fitness girl emerging who had finished with wallowing at rock bottom. She was ready to go to any lengths to pursue her athletic dreams. Reckless fitness girl was trying to break free while my old self was trying to take cover. As my two identities grappled, I was gripped by a tug of war between fear and excitement for change—but eventually reckless fitness girl triumphed and began to occupy my being.

As the start date for 5K training drew near, my anxiety mounted. My heart raced, my breathing was labored, and the tension in my shoulders was almost unbearable. What if I was the biggest? The slowest? What if I couldn't keep up? But reckless fitness girl wouldn't listen to the negative voice desperately trying to convince her to stay home. She pushed through, and I arrived there that first night, determined to try even if I felt like an imposter in my running clothes. I tried to look self-assured among the "real" runners. I'm sure I reeked of fear and self-consciousness, but it was all secondary to the churning emotions I felt about my debut at my new run club.

JUST AS I was about to take my seat among the runners crowding the store, a woman stood up in front of us and introduced herself as our run leader. When I turned my gaze toward her, I was shocked to see a plus-size woman decked out in running gear. Her name was Chris. When I looked at her, I saw an icon, a rock star, and a total game-changer. My crippling fear melted away; I was not alone. That night, as we hit the streets for our first run, I caught a glimpse of what was possible. Not only did I make it through the run (and not die!), but on the way home I couldn't stop smiling. Chris never mentioned body size or weight loss. We were all athletes to her, on a mission to run hard, run strong, and run for healthy outcomes. Her passion for running was inspiring, and she taught me that by showing up and being there that first day, I was the only thing holding me back. I am here to share that message with you now.

You are capable of anything you set your mind to.

I started to find other examples of plus-size women accomplishing kick-ass feats in fitness who, along with Chris, fed my sense of belonging and helped me stay motivated. Jayne Williams, author of *Slow Fat Triathlete,* was working her way through the triathlon circuit and becoming a strong voice for women of size in the triathlon community. Cheryl Haworth was rocking the weightlifting events at the 2000 Summer

Olympics and went on to become a three-time Olympian. The more I looked around, the more I noticed women of size standing up and participating.

Despite this, I still wanted to lose weight, but this desire took a backseat to the rewards of my physical achievements. I observed other plus-size women being recognized for their athleticism, and recognized the same potential in myself. We still have a long way to go, but the media are starting to wake up to examples of athletes just like you and me. Plus-size women are competing at the Olympics in weightlifting and track and field. They're playing soccer, and they're running triathlons and marathons. They're training at fitness classes all around the world.

Throughout history, our plus-size male counterparts have been more visible, performing at elite levels in the NFL, in the boxing ring, and on the PGA tour. This is not a new concept. Plus-size athletes appear throughout Japanese history in sumo wrestling, the country's national sport. In sumo, the bigger the body, the bigger the advantage and the more power behind the grapple.

When I opened my eyes and took a closer look, I found plus-size athletes in small pockets throughout society. This discovery was the beginning of my belief that big bodies can also be fit and athletic bodies. My entire outlook on what was possible changed dramatically. In my mind, the size of my body was no longer a barrier to becoming an athlete, and I started to feel unstoppable. Your body size is not a barrier for you either. You too can be unstoppable.

I began running regularly, and with a few races under my belt, I ventured into cross-training. I hired a personal trainer, Amanda, to support me as I learned how to lift weights. Like Chris, she never treated me differently because of my body size. She pushed me to become more and more of an athlete.

After several months of working together, she asked me if I wanted to help her as a run leader for a "Learn to Run 10K" clinic. After running for a few years, I was now in the position to be just like Chris: to inspire and lead new runners to their first finish line. The old, frightened me wanted to say no. The new, reckless fitness girl said, "Hell yes!"

The next thirteen weeks were the most rewarding of my life as I helped lead a group of people to their first 10K race. On the day of the race, I guided the group through sun and rain; we ran like warriors who couldn't be stopped. Not long before, I had been where they were, and I knew what they were feeling—a combination of worry, doubt, and hope. On race day I reflected on how far I had come and was grateful I had allowed myself to pay it forward. From that moment, I was hooked on leading others to achieve their athletic dreams. From there it was a short path to becoming a certified fitness professional, quitting my unfulfilling day job, and creating an innovative fitness company geared toward helping plus-size women achieve their athletic dreams.

Whether you are an avid walker, a triathlete, a ballroom dancer, or an Olympic weightlifter, or if you aspire to be all these things and more, your presence as a plus-size woman working out in our society is creating a much-needed shift. And because we don't see women of size as much as we need to in advertising, television, movies, or other media, it's up to us—you and me—to inspire others to join our ranks.

Athletes come in all shapes and sizes. Everyone needs to know this. When society as a whole starts to recognize plus-size athleticism as something real and measurable, the resulting profound social shift will improve the lives of everybody. People will become less judgmental, more women will engage in physical exercise, and their fear of gym culture will be reduced. If members of the plus-size community could see themselves represented in sports and athletics, our world would change dramatically—for the better.

Since the day I walked into my first running clinic fifteen years ago, I have trained and interacted with thousands of plus-size women. I've helped them realize their athletic potential simply by showing up and giving back what was given to me. I see amazing fitness feats from women of all shapes and sizes and I love watching their own reckless fitness girl emerge and take over. It is equally gratifying to watch their mindset change from diet girl to Big Fit Girl. I know that they are unstoppable and limitless—and you can be too.

I am living proof that this true. I found a different approach to fitness, and it changed my life. Ever since, I've committed my life as a trainer with my own fitness business to showing women of size how to reach their athletic dreams. Through my own story, personal profiles of other Big Fit Girls, and tips for how to live an athletic life, I hope to inspire you to stop feeling that success is only possible when you are thin, to embrace the body you are in, and to make your fitness goals a reality—to be seen more, to sweat more, and to conquer more.

HERE ARE SOME of the things you will find in this book:

1. Real women living their athletic dreams: Stories of women changing their lives, creating a limitless way of life, and achieving their athletic goals.
2. Body politics: A look at the fundamental social and psychological reasons why people struggle to make fitness a part of their daily lives. Knowledge is power; you'll get that here!
3. Practical fitness advice: Practical fitness and body love tips geared toward the plus-size woman. It's about time someone wrote something just for us Big Fit Girls.
4. Inspirational messages from leading plus-size women:

Advice from plus-size Olympians, fitness professionals, TV personalities, bloggers, and fitness enthusiasts.

5. A cultural education: An examination of Western cultural ideals and how they affect the choice to be limitless or limited in our lives.

6. Fitness gear talk: An extensive list of the best fitness gear for plus-size athletes that includes advice on where to get it so that you can live your athletic dreams in comfort and with confidence.

7. Recipe for an active lifestyle, long term: Advice on how to stop jumping on and off the wagon and make fitness a lifestyle for good.

8. Nutrition talk, not diet talk: A discussion on how to nurture your body for your best athletic performance without measuring, counting points, or restricting what you eat—just healthy food in abundance. Food is not the enemy!

9. How to find the right fitness professional: An introduction to the art of finding the right people to help you stay fit for the long term.

10. A 5K training plan for plus-size athletes: A practical and doable plan for your busy life. After training thousands of plus-size women, I know what works and what doesn't. The 5K distance is a great place to start. The plan is easy to follow, you can either walk or learn to run the distance, it's free, and training can be done at any time of the day. The accomplishment is extremely measurable and will give you the inspiration and confidence to continue in your fitness journey.

11. A fitness glossary: The language, terminology, and non-verbal cues that come with many fitness environments can often leave you feeling like a fish out of water. I've outlined all you need to know so that you never have to feel lost as you work to achieve your athletic goals.

I ALSO SHARE my personal experiences, from my darkest hours to my greatest victories. My growing list of achievements kept pushing me forward to build the athletic lifestyle I had dreamed of for years. I hope that this book will help you to do the same.

# ONE

# Shattering Stereotypes

I RAN MY FIRST half-marathon in San Francisco. When I woke up on race day, my stomach was churning with both fear and excitement. Getting ready in front of the mirror that morning, I repeated my mantra: *You are an athlete. You are a champion who has put in the training time. You belong here.*

When I arrived at the race location and caught my first glimpse of the start line for the 30th Annual Kaiser Permanente Half Marathon and 5K, I felt even more determined. This was the beginning of one of the most demanding days of my life, and I was filled with excitement and growing confidence. As I approached the desk to pick up my race package, I caught the eye of the young man behind the table. He asked my name and without hesitation reached for the 5K race package. He assumed I was participating in the (much) shorter race.

This moment speaks volumes about how people perceive those of us with larger bodies and why many of us feel that we don't fit in. My body size communicated to him that I was not physically capable of running the event's longer race. This happens at most events I participate in: someone might make an out-of-line comment or show surprise or express an assumption about what my body is capable of. The same thing happens when I tell people that I am a personal trainer and I own a fitness business.

"I am here to run the half-marathon," I said sharply. "Oh," he said, quickly fumbling for my race package in the other box. I took my number and the event-branded race shirt that was three sizes too small and joined my husband.

The little voice inside cheering me on had been reduced to a whisper. As we stood silently waiting for the race to begin, I couldn't help feeling defeated. I had trained for months and run hundreds of miles, and yet this encounter left me feeling like an impostor. I had felt this before—like I didn't fit in.

Unfortunately, this feeling of sitting on the sidelines can be common among women of size who participate in races; perhaps you have felt this way too. Throughout my career as a trainer, women have shared stories of fitness classes, races, and high school gym classes where their potential was repeatedly overlooked because of their size. As humans, we crave acceptance. And these memories of rejection linger and hold us back.

## Identity Threat and Stereotypes

DR. BRENDA MAJOR is a professor of psychology at the University of California, Santa Barbara. Major's research focuses on how people cope with prejudice and discrimination. She confirms what I've noted from teaching fitness to plus-size women: the fear of judgment is real and often warranted.

"Evidence around stigma, discrimination, and negative attitudes is incredibly strong," says Major, "and people are aware of these judgments by others. In my primary discipline—social psychology—I've studied 'social identity threat' at length, which is an awareness that other people are judging you and seeing you negatively on the basis of the identities you have, in this case being fat, which is a severely devalued identity in America. As a result, many of us internalize these judgments as our own. We not only feel negatively judged by others, but we judge ourselves. There's this very strong and real fear that you are going to be negatively evaluated and excluded."

Major's findings explain a lot about why many people find fitness unapproachable. When we feel judged by others, our fear and anxiety grows. For this reason, many of us find fitness endeavors intimidating and out of reach.

Though we may not have the power to change others' judgments, we can change this dynamic—the key lies in our response. If you are feeling judged, you can take control of the situation. Often when people judge others, it's because of their own feelings of inadequacy. Know that their judgments are their issues, not yours. It can be difficult to do this, but take pride in your sense of self and try to stay confident and true to your athletic dreams.

Experts say that the way we confront bias and discrimination often depends on the situation and the personality type of the individual being judged. Research shows that bias toward and discrimination against people who are fat most often comes from physicians and family members. If you feel you can, take a stand against them. It doesn't have to be confrontational or abrasive. For example, if a family member is harping on you to lose weight you could say, "I appreciate your concern for my health, but I am working on my health in a way that works for me." Rehearse your response and advocate for yourself. And if that fails, step away. Although we can never escape all bias, especially from our family members, when it comes to judgments about our weight, we can remove ourselves from harmful situations. Find people who support you, and avoid those who don't.

It may also help to practice compassion toward people who judge you. Holding on to resentment and anger will only hurt you. Creating a toolbox of skills and strategies to cope with bias toward those who are fat has helped me understand the knee-jerk reaction of that young man behind the table on race day. His action was fueled by a culture that has one narrative about bodies and health. Eventually, I felt only compassion for him. How could I blame him for his assumptions about me?

While many people assume that fat automatically equals unfit, a growing number of highly respected researchers and agencies say otherwise. Dr. Steven Blair is a renowned exercise researcher at the Arnold School of Public Health at the University of South Carolina. His research shows that excess weight is not "the enemy." Not getting enough exercise and being cardiovascularly unfit are much greater contributors to poor health than any extra pounds can be. Blair stands firmly by his research showing that fit, fat people outlive thin, unfit people. The National Cancer Institute also backed this finding, reporting that physical activity is associated with greater longevity among persons in all BMI groups: those normal weight, and those considered fat.

Although many studies demonstrate that a fit body can come in a range of sizes, many people can't see beyond the stereotypes. Larger bodies seldom appear in advertisements for gyms or in fitness magazines. When we do see a fat body in the media, it often accompanies an article about the latest demonizing obesity study and shows the person from only the shoulders down, dehumanizing the person. Athletes like me who fall outside of the athletic norm often feel we don't fit in because we've been told, in subtle and not-so-subtle ways, that we don't.

Changing our fitness experience means surrounding ourselves with positive influences and finding teams of people who leave stereotypes at the door. And because we seldom see athletes of size in our daily visual landscape, it's up to you and me to change the perceptions out there.

THERE ARE A number of things we can all do to shatter stereotypes surrounding people of size and show society a new version of the plus-size woman:

1. Sign up for a 5K walk or run. Being seen participating in sporting events makes a powerful statement: plus-size does not mean inactive, unfit, or unhealthy. The more people like you and me who are seen at such events, the more our participation will be perceived as normal.

2. Perhaps you have a bucket list but felt you needed to be thinner or more fit to do these things you've always wanted to do. Jump out of a plane? Do an obstacle mud race? I always wanted to hike to the bottom of the Grand Canyon— so I did! Today is a gift and tomorrow is not guaranteed, so start ticking off the boxes.

3. Don't wait for someday—live your life on your terms today. Maybe going to the beach is something you've been waiting to do when you are thinner? Everyone deserves to swim and enjoy the beach. I love the saying, "If you have a body and you go to the beach, you have a beach body!" You *can* rock a bathing suit. Buy one that makes you feel good and then strut your stuff. There is more than one type of bathing suit body. (See the gear section of this book for great retailers in swimwear.)

4. Wear what you want. Try something that is out of your comfort zone but that you've always wanted to wear: bold prints, fitted clothing, and horizontal stripes come to mind. Bodies of size do not need to be all covered up, draped in black, or restricted to plain clothing. Wear what makes you feel good.

5. Accept yourself. Abandoning diet culture and rocking the body you have shatters the stereotype that all big women are on a mission to become thin. And, in case you haven't heard, you don't have to be on that mission anymore.

THERE IS A misconception that people like us are crying into our pillows every night wishing we could lose weight and find happiness. But your weight should not determine your happiness. Live your happiest life now, not when you are thinner. Show yourself and the world that big girls rule their lives.

**Sarah Robles, Olympic weightlifter, Team USA 2012 and 2016:**
"I think limits are only put on us by ourselves. People can say or feel any way about us and place caps on our abilities, but we are the ones who choose how we react and if we put those limits on ourselves. To be limitless is the ultimate freedom to choose our destiny. Had I put caps on what I could do or who I could be, I wouldn't be living the amazing life I am. I get to do what I love with people I love and help others because I chose a limitless path, one very few have traversed."

Stacey Williams exemplifies this idea. A plus-size athlete from Dallas, Texas, she started her athletic journey as an unhealthy and unhappy woman.

"I didn't know where to start," she says. "I felt so intimidated to change my life but I desperately wanted to change. Going to the gym just felt too scary because I thought people would laugh at me. No one at the gym looked like me; everyone looked like they were already fit."

Stacey started exercising at home using fitness DVDs. "It was the only way I could exercise and feel comfortable doing it. I just didn't have the confidence to do it in public."

Because of her size, Stacey didn't feel that she belonged in a conventional gym. So she started walking on her own in her neighborhood. At first she walked ten minutes a day. She gradually worked up to twenty minutes a day and then thirty. Six months later she was walking one to two hours each day and had never felt stronger.

Stacey built her strength and her confidence up enough to join a walking group at a local club in her neighborhood; now she is training for a half-marathon walk.

I wish all gyms were welcoming places for everyone, regardless of size, but by getting out there and getting involved in fitness, wherever you feel comfortable, your participation shatters all the stereotypes that big women face.

## How the Media Play a Role in Creating Stereotypes

ALTHOUGH STATISTICALLY, APPROXIMATELY 67 percent of North American women are a size 14 or larger,[1] we don't see ourselves represented in the media. Plus-size women are an invisible majority. When we don't see ourselves, many of us conclude that we don't belong.

By the time she is twelve, the average American girl has seen over 77,000 commercials. American teenagers consume ten hours and forty-five minutes of media every day through the Internet, television, music, movies, and magazines. What does this mean for young women? During this vital stage of life they are highly impressionable, and the impression they get isn't good. Young girls are bombarded with images of tall, very thin girls with tanned skin and blonde hair, and if they don't recognize themselves in these images it opens the door to feelings of failure. Our communities and families do not always provide girls their first role models; in many cases mass media have taken over. By the time they're teenagers, if girls cannot see their likeness in this onslaught of messaging, they may begin to feel isolated and abnormal. These feelings are built on a foundation of never measuring up, failing to achieve an ideal, and not being good enough.

Until recently, mass media have rarely presented larger women in a positive way. Negative stories about larger bodies are fodder for headlines.

- "Lawyer Sues Airline for Having to Sit Next to Obese Passenger" (*The Independent*, September 23, 2016)
- "Obesity Rates Reach Historic Highs in Most U.S. States" (NBC News, September 4, 2014)
- "Teen Tennis Player Brings Weight to French Open" (*Daily Mail*, September 7, 2012)

Many publications celebrate one image of fitness rather than championing diversity in size among athletes. Not surprisingly, the population at large doesn't associate health and athletics with larger bodies. We've become so used to seeing very thin bodies as the norm that it's distorted our ideas of what is average. It's why people like comedian Amy Schumer are labeled "plus-size" by the media when Schumer at most is a size 10.

The average size of most models featured on the cover of fitness magazines is size 2 to 4. This means that major fitness magazines do not represent nearly 70 percent of North American women; the exclusion is a social injustice.

Things are changing. I see it every day; the mere fact that this book has been published is another push back against the oppression of larger women. The fitness industry is becoming more inclusive and body positive. It has no choice: people are demanding it.

In August 2015, for the first time in its history, *Women's Running* magazine made the bold move of featuring plus-size athlete Erica Schenk on its cover. In the photo, young and vibrant Schenk runs confidently down a park path looking like an experienced runner in her running tights and rose-colored athletic tank top. Her big body looks powerful as she gazes into the distance. She runs with a smile, exuding freedom. She looks like a natural-born athlete.

On the *Today* show, *Women's Running* editor-in-chief Jessica Sebor spoke about her motive behind the cover. "There's a stereotype that all runners are skinny," Sebor said. "And that's just not the case. Runners come in all shapes and sizes. You can go to any race finish line, from a 5K to a marathon, and see that. It was important for us to celebrate that."

Sport England completed a survey of women between the ages of fourteen and forty and found that two million fewer British women play sports than British men. But 75 percent of those women want to be active but aren't out of fear of judgment.

Based on their findings, in January 2015, Sport England launched the highly successful "This Girl Can" campaign, which beautifully showcased size diversity in fitness and sport to inspire women to "wiggle, jiggle, move, and prove that judgment is a barrier that can be overcome." Using regular women in the campaign, they posted large ads throughout Britain showing women working out in all their "un-Photoshopped" glory. Like *Women's Running*, Sport England's campaign became an international news sensation.

When we show diversity, we get diversity. Sport England reported that since celebrating the first birthday of the "This Girl Can" campaign, women of all shapes, sizes, ages, and ethnicities are getting active in greater numbers. A study showed that 2.8 million British women have increased their physical activity since viewing the groundbreaking campaign. "This Girl Can" has sparked conversations in 110 countries worldwide, and more than 540,000 women and girls have joined their online community. The campaign's popularity keeps growing and the videos and images have been viewed more than 40 million times through various social media.

Could this be the start of a new wave in media and advertising? Positive representation of diversely sized athletes is the key to the future of women of size in sports. When we see ourselves pictured in magazines, on television, and in advertisements, we feel invited, inspired, and motivated to join in.

Visual imagery strongly drives human thought patterns, and it currently excludes plus-size women in a big way. Media that depicts women of size is essential to changing the image of plus-size women. But there's good news: we can create change and dictate what we want through what we choose to consume. Long ago, I decided to strip down my media consumption and avoid unhealthy images and messages of women. I removed media that portrayed women inaccurately from my newsfeed, bookmarks, and magazine racks. I started following body-positive leaders and brands that were spreading a new, positive message for women and girls. I stopped buying overly Photoshopped fashion and fitness magazines and started to invite only positive imagery into my sightline. I took control. Now, I dictate what I see. It's not possible to hide everything that doesn't speak to you, but if we refuse to buy in to exclusionary messaging, brands and media will be forced to change their strategies.

If we work together, we can create change. Take the healthy media pledge with me! Use the hashtag #healthymediapledge and share it with your sisters, mother, daughters, and friends.

*I pledge to ditch negative media from my news feed, email inbox, and magazine stack. I will no longer consume media that doesn't celebrate who I am. #healthymediapledge*

## How Athletic Branding Impacts Stereotypes

CONVENTIONAL ATHLETIC BRANDS don't design their products for a diverse range of body sizes. Major brands steer clear of larger-bodied representatives, deepening the misconception that bigger bodies can't be athletic or healthy.

At the height of the 2012 Summer Olympics and Nike's "Find Your Greatness" campaign, the activewear brand released a commercial called "The Jogger." The commercial featured a 232-pound twelve-year-old boy named Nathan Sorrell. The ad was nicknamed "Fat Boy Running" on social media.

The commercial was powerful in its simplicity, showing uncut footage of Sorrell jogging down a long, empty road, breathing hard but persevering. A calm voice narrated: "Greatness. It's just something we made up. Somehow we've come to believe that greatness is a gift reserved for a chosen few. For prodigies. For superstars. And the rest of us can only stand by watching. You can forget that. Greatness is not some rare DNA strand. It's not some precious thing. Greatness is no more unique to us than breathing. We're all capable of it. All of us."

The ad struck a chord with millions of people. Even though Nike wasn't an official Olympic sponsor, the spot stole the show—as did young Nathan.

Despite its popularity—the video has 1.7 million views on YouTube—this campaign remains one of the very few instances where a larger body has been associated with a major athletic brand. Clearly the numbers show we want more! We need more examples of diversity in size from brand names. We must continue to celebrate magazines, companies, and campaigns that bravely step away from misleading cultural norms and include all shapes and sizes in their messaging and mission.

Only we can drive that change. Brands respond to trends, commerce, and demand, so it's up to us—you and me—to take a stand against brands that represent only one ideal body size. Join me in changing athletic brand culture to include body size diversity.

Use the hashtag #brandmysize with pictures of yourself and other women of size on your social feeds.

*I pledge to buy only athletic apparel from brands that not only cater to my size but also show women of my size in their marketing and advertising. #brandmysize*

## How Advertising Impacts Stereotypes

"ADVERTISING IS MUCH more than ads. It sells values, images, concepts of love, sexuality and success and perhaps most important, normalcy. To a great extent it tells us who we are and who we should be," says Jean Kilbourne, renowned lecturer whose work is the focus of the documentary *Killing Us Softly: Advertising's Image of Women.*

But there is hope: behind closed doors at advertising agencies around the world, the percentage of female creative directors is growing (from 3 percent to 11 percent in the last three years), an increase that has the potential to change the face of advertising. When more women are shaping media, they are likely to expand how women are represented, with more diversity and accuracy.

Jean Batthany, a creative director at one of the world's leading advertising agencies, is pushing for gender equality in the advertising world. "Women make up only 11 percent of creative directors in the United States," she says. "Yet women make, on average, 85 percent of purchase decisions in the home. The hope is that if more women are leading the creative charge, the messages and images can and will be even more representative and persuasive to women. And that's just good business."

Batthany continues, "With men as the majority, women are viewed and portrayed through the male gaze. More specifically, it's the idea that films and advertisements were created to please a heterosexual male audience."

In most advertising, plus-size women are invisible; we simply don't exist. Batthany sees things slowly changing, however; some advertisers are now coming to the table to talk not only about their products but also about their social mission.

"I definitely feel a shift as of late. This year there was lots of buzz when a *Sports Illustrated* swimsuit issue featured a plus-size model for the first time. Truth be told, it was a paid ad for Swimsuits for All featuring drop-dead gorgeous and sexy-as-hell plus-model Ashley Graham, and it got people talking!"

APPROXIMATELY 108 MILLION American women are size 14 or larger, and yet they remain virtually invisible in advertising and media. Though diversity in representation is on the rise, seeing a plus-size woman portrayed positively or shown in a position of power in advertisements is still rare.

Batthany says that although the Internet leads to faster change, cultural shifts take time. "Knowing the power of mass media, I am constantly reminding my two extremely self-conscious teenage daughters that the images they are exposed to are not real. They are retouched, edited, manipulated. It takes a village of hairstylists, makeup artists, wardrobe stylists, lighting specialists, cinematographers, photographers, and editors to get that one seemingly perfect shot. I have seen first-hand how self-esteem can be damaged by not fitting 'the norm.' Body hating, body shaming, eating disorders, and depression feel like they are at epidemic levels."

"The good news," she says, "is there definitely seems to be a movement toward redefining what is beautiful. And I am a firm believer in the adage 'you cannot be what you do not see.'"

Together, let's push to see more, so we can all be more. If companies and advertisers are hit in the pocketbook, they will be forced to make the change. Take the pledge and join me in creating important social change.

*I pledge to eliminate or reduce my purchases of products from brands with harmful advertising messages or advertisers that alter the bodies and appearance of women in their advertisements. I pledge to use my purchasing power to support brands that promote healthy bodies and include women of all shapes and sizes in their messages.*

## How the Diet Industry Impacts Stereotypes

IF YOU ARE like me, you've probably tried to diet many times to conform to the ideal body type portrayed by the media. Disliking your body or feeling shame about it can prevent you from realizing your dreams and your fitness goals. The weight-loss industry offers empty promises of a new you and a better life. In the checkout line at most grocery stores magazine headlines tempt female shoppers to try the latest gimmick:

- "Look Hotter Naked" (*Cosmopolitan*, February 2016)
- "Better than Lap Band, Lose 25 lbs. in 8 Weeks" (*Woman's World*, January 2014)
- "Your Dream Body in Just 2 Weeks" (*Shape*, January 2016)

Don't buy in! We all know from experience that these "solutions" don't solve any of our problems.

Melissa A. Fabello, a body-positive activist, sexuality scholar, and managing editor at *Everyday Feminism,* is critical of how plus-size women are perceived and treated in our weight loss–driven culture. "Currently, what's on trend is for women to be thin but curvy, but not *fat* curvy. As we create narrower and narrower beauty standards, we create more and more disdain for anyone who falls, really, on either side of that ideal. However, the way that we look at ultra-thin bodies versus ultra-lush bodies is very different. We understand ultra-thin bodies as the embodiment of the constructs of 'control' and 'willpower' that diet culture sells us. And we understand fat bodies as the exact opposite—as a manifestation of sloth and gluttony."

The annual revenue of the U.S. weight-loss industry—including diet books, diet drugs, and weight-loss surgeries—is 20 billion dollars. This staggering figure reveals how much desperation women feel; we will do anything to attain the feminine ideal, and marketers sell us on their unproven solution: weight loss.

*We* aren't defective; the system is defective.

---

**Jillian Camarena-Williams, Olympic shot-putter, Team USA 2008 and 2012:** "'Healthy' means taking care of your body both physically and mentally. Too many people want to lose weight or change their body. I once did a Dexa scan, a scan that tells you your body composition. If I had 0 percent body fat I would still have weighed 170 lbs. That is still not a small girl. I knew I was taking care of my body, exercising, eating healthfully, and my body felt good. I may not have been my 'ideal' weight, but my body was healthy and functioning properly and that was all I could do!"

---

When I realized that my weight didn't have to be a barrier to my happiness, I let go of chasing thinness. Ironically, this made me happier. I abandoned dieting and decided to pursue my athletic dreams in the body I had. My fitness goals were no longer about burning calories but about challenging myself, persevering, and achieving victory through the goals I set for myself.

## How to Be the Change and Shatter Stereotypes

WHILE NOT ALWAYS easy, adhering to the following principles will help you ignore the influence of biased media. These suggestions have worked for me on my journey to athleticism and self-love:

### CONSUME AND SHARE MEDIA THAT ACCURATELY DEPICT WOMEN IN A RANGE OF SIZES

Diverse images of women are starting to appear more frequently, as we've seen with Erica Schenk's cover of *Women's Running* and the "This Girl Can" campaign. Other examples include the July 2015 cover of ESPN *The Magazine,* featuring plus-size Olympian Amanda Bingson in the nude. In 2016, for the first time in the magazine's history, *Sports Illustrated* featured a plus-size model, Ashley Graham, on its cover, and the iconic brand Nike included diversity in their Brahaus Collection advertising by featuring plus-size model Paloma Elsesser. When you see images and stories like these, share the hell out of them on your social networks. Start conversations about size diversity in sports. Get to know the game-changers who are out there leading the way—it can change the way you think about your own body and athleticism. But in order to do that, you need to know where to find them. With that in mind, here are seven places to find body-positive and size-friendly media:

1. *My Name Is Jessamyn*
   Jessamyn Stanley is a yoga teacher, body-positive advocate, and writer from Durham, North Carolina. Stanley

has gathered a significant following documenting her yoga journey on Tumblr and Instagram.
jessamynstanley.com

2. Body Positive Athletes
According to their website, "Body Positive Athletes is a community of people who believe that the term 'athletic' defines a lifestyle and not a body shape or size. We represent people from all walks of life—coaches, athletes, trainers, and people who simply enjoy pursuing a healthy lifestyle. We have a common goal of celebrating the function of the body and the diversity of physiques in sport."
bodypositiveathletes.wordpress.com

3. *FabUplus Magazine*
*FabUplus Magazine* is the long-awaited voice of the plus-size community. As North America's first body-positive health, fitness, and lifestyle magazine with weight neutral content dedicated to women with curves, *FabUplus* is breaking traditional media rules by showcasing women of size and encouraging women to be confident.
fabuplusmagazine.com

4. "This Girl Can" Campaign
"This Girl Can" is a national campaign developed by Sport England alongside a wide range of partnership organizations. It's a celebration of active women throughout England who are doing their thing no matter how well they do it, how they look, or even how red their faces get.
thisgirlcan.co.uk

5. *The Militant Baker*
*The Militant Baker* is a popular blog authored by Jes Baker.

Baker covers a mixture of subjects ranging from the delightful to the very uncomfortable. Her topics include the hazardous journey of body acceptance, how to take boudoir photos, and general empowerment. Baker's wit and humor can also be found in her book, *Things No One Will Tell Fat Girls*.

themilitantbaker.com

6. Adios Barbie

Since the dawn of the web (or at least since 1998), feminist site adiosbarbie.com has been on a mission to broaden the discussion of body image to include race, gender, sexual orientation, dis/ability, age, and size.

adiosbarbie.com

7. About-Face

About-Face is an educational website whose vision is for women and girls to lead full lives, unconstrained by preoccupations with appearance and body image. It also aims for gender-balanced and gender-neutral media representation. The website offers tools and workshops to create change for women and girls.

about-face.org

**BE THE MEDIA!**

In the social media era, we all have a platform to share our views. Jes Baker became a well-known body-positive advocate when she rebutted Abercrombie & Fitch's CEO, Mike Jeffries, who had publicly stated that his company only makes clothes for smaller women (as he called them, "cool kids"); they intentionally do not sell larger sizes. Baker, a plus-size woman, took striking photos of herself posing with a conventionally hot male model and used them to create the "Attractive & Fat" campaign, which played on the branding and typography used in Abercrombie & Fitch's advertising. This campaign landed Baker on the *Today* show, and her story was covered by most international media outlets. Baker is proof that if no one is doing it for you, you can definitely make a statement on your own terms.

## FIND SUPPORTIVE HEALTH AND FITNESS ENVIRONMENTS

Finding your fit in fitness is an important component of your continued success. Look for gyms, leaders, and trainers who support body-positive training, and who are not hyper-focused on weight loss. In my own experience, the people who believed in my goals without casting judgment or asking me to change my body became essential to my journey. These types of people and environments are usually behind the doors of gyms that represent you and me. Look for gyms that embody who you are in their marketing. Ask yourself these questions: Does their website show a range of sizes, ages, and ethnicities? Are they giving you the unspoken invitation to join the gym in their marketing by demonstrating that their services are for you? Gyms that *do* represent you have carefully thought this through and have emphasized inclusiveness in their messaging. This communicates a lot before you've even walked in the door. This gym is ready for you.

## PARTICIPATE IN ATHLETICS IN YOUR COMMUNITY

I know how hard it is, at first, to show up for the race or the dance class. But when you do, you represent size diversity and send an important message to the others present. Many people have never seen people with larger bodies kicking ass in athletics. Your appearance tells a new story that is revolutionary. You will feel empowered, and others will be encouraged.

Recently I spoke to a large group of plus-size women on the topic of athleticism at every size. When I brought up the subject of participation and how representing size diversity can influence others to join in, a woman proudly put her hand up and told me that a while ago she very reluctantly started dance classes. She was doing the type of dance that you see on *Dancing with the Stars* and was getting quite good at it. That soon progressed into local competitions; all the while she was having a ball doing it (no pun intended). She said someone would often approach her after the competition and tell her how much she had inspired them to get active. Seeing is believing in yourself, and until we see bigger bodies in fitness media and advertising, it really is up to you and me to spread the word and be the change.

### CREATE A SPACE OF NO NEGATIVE BODY TALK

Women often deflect compliments by saying something negative about themselves. I have been guilty of this too. Someone might say, "Your hair looks great today," and often my reaction would be something like, "Really? I haven't washed it or styled it in two days." Turning a positive comment into something negative was habitual for me until I became more self-aware.

The pursuit of perfection is so ingrained in us that we say things about ourselves that we would never say to another woman. When people compliment you, accept the compliment with a smile. When negative thoughts enter your mind, push them out with something positive. With love and kindness, call others out on their own negative self-talk. An example might be when a friend says "I look terrible today," to respond by saying, "No you don't. We can't always look amazing and we are more than our looks. Words really matter, so be kind to yourself!" Avoid gossiping about others, too. Often our criticism of others is a reflection of how we feel about ourselves. Women need to support each other more and champion what makes each of us unique. Start doing this today, in all areas of your life.

Here is the strategy that helped me change my thought patterns. Have you ever been in a department store to return an item and observed the cashier calling over the manager to override the transaction? I want you to be the manager of your mind. I want you to override your negative self-talk. Have you heard the saying, "Fake it till you make it"? You might have to fake it at first. As soon as a negative thought comes into your mind, like "Man, I look fat in these shorts, why did I leave the house looking like this"—that is when you call in the manager for an override.

When you override, you deflect and retort with something more positive. "These shorts are great and show off my strong legs" is an example, but say whatever feels authentically positive about yourself. Over time you'll train your brain and the override will be needed less and less until your thinking is mostly positive. It takes time, but it works. Take control; you are your mind's manager.

### REJECT WEIGHT-LOSS CULTURE AND PERFECTIONISM

We need to quit trying to attain what society deems the perfect body and instead create our own ideals based on what feels good to us. All bodies are good bodies, and most of us just don't have the same genetics as the models we see in magazines. In fact, only a very small number of women do. We need to embrace and celebrate who we are, as we are.

Melissa A. Fabello speaks to this beautifully: "I think that perfectionism is dangerous—and I say this as a recovering perfectionist! I think that we've created an environment in which we expect 'the best' from people, but we define what is 'best' for them. We don't allow people to be their happiest, healthiest selves. Instead, we impose a one-size-fits-all cultural standard of 'ideal' on them, and we reinforce that by celebrating those who reach it and denigrating those who can't."

## RECOGNIZE YOUR OWN AND OUR COLLECTIVE POWER

Alice Walker, author of *The Color Purple,* eloquently describes the potential power of a collective group: "The most common way people give up their power is by thinking they don't have any."

We *do* have the power to create change. We have the power to stand up and say that women of size can be athletes, leaders, and advocates. We can love our bodies and be valued women, regardless of our size. We are worthy.

When we demand that publications, companies, and advertisers reflect our ideals in their messages, they will do so. After all, these businesses are driven by the market; they give us what we want! Let's want something that benefits us. Because magazine editors now know that there's a substantial audience that, until recently, has been ignored, we're beginning to see plus-size women becoming cover girls. The fashion industry can no longer overlook the buying power of millions of plus-size women and have started to step up and deliver larger sizes at many mainstream retailers.

Awareness gives us the power to change and the ability to kick open the door to living limitlessly. And together, through efforts large and small, we can shatter stereotypes and change the world.

## TAKE THE BODY POSITIVE PLEDGE

Taking the body positive pledge is a great way to commit to your new way of thinking. It takes time to unlearn everything that you have learned, so let's get started now. We are bombarded by images and messages telling us that we don't belong. We must stop believing this and fight to be respected and included as we are. Let's make it official:

*I promise to love and respect my body every day. I recognize that not every moment will include body love, but I am committed to changing my thought patterns and inviting body love and self-acceptance into my life.*

*Through this process I vow to (to the best of my ability):*

- *Start my morning with affirmations about something I love about myself.*
- *Refrain from negative self-talk.*
- *Live my life to its fullest in the body I have now.*
- *Say "yes" more than "no" to things that scare me.*
- *Refrain from thinking or saying negative things about myself or other people.*
- *Ditch negative media.*
- *Surround myself with positive people who only elevate me.*
- *Accept compliments graciously.*

*On the days when this seems impossible, I will be kind to myself and keep in mind that this is a journey. Things don't change overnight. Tomorrow is a new day. It's time to shatter the stereotypes in my life and be the change.*

# TWO

# Unleashing Your Inner Athlete

I AM AN ATHLETE. When I run the streets of my neighborhood with my running tribe around me, pushing my body to its limits, sweat dripping from my forehead, I am an athlete. When I race across the finish line, swim my final lap, or finish a particularly challenging fitness class, I am an athlete. And you can become an athlete too.

In the past I tried many times to find my way to an active life. Maybe you can relate: I would start an activity only to get discouraged and end up back on the couch, feeling guilty and defeated. I would be overly enthusiastic and join a new gym, commit myself to a two-year contract, and vow that this time I would finally get my shit together. I would shift excessively into "all" mode and then in fairly short order slip back into "nothing" mode, then add up more failure and disappointment.

I was convinced, and maybe you are too, that athletics and the healthful life I desired were reserved for a group of thin elites. Why was I convinced that I could only be an athlete if I fit a particular body type?

"Athlete," as defined by the *Oxford English Dictionary*, means a person who is proficient in fitness or sport. Proficient. *Oxford* does not mention age, gender, race, or physical size. Today, by society's standards, the word "athlete" means being ripped and muscular. When men or women fit the dictionary definition of "athlete" but do not have the body type dictated by our culture, they may be subject to ridicule.

You may remember what the reaction was to baseball player Prince Fielder when his fat, naked body graced the cover of ESPN *The Magazine* in 2014. The Internet exploded with body-shaming comments that ridiculed Fielder for his strong, muscular—but apparently not ripped enough—physique. We are guilty, collectively, of associating "athlete" with thin, muscular frames but not bodies that fall outside of that narrow range.

At a press conference Fielder spoke his truth about the reaction from society. "A lot of people probably think I'm not athletic or don't even try to work out or whatever, but I do," Fielder said. "Just because you're big doesn't mean you can't be an athlete. And, just because you work out doesn't mean you're going to have a twelve-pack. I work out to make sure I can do my job to the best of my ability. Other than that, I'm not going up there trying to be a fitness model."

It's time to restore the true meaning of the word "athlete." Everyone has the ability to become athletically proficient, to achieve and often exceed their expectations of themselves, and everyone has the right to bring their bad-ass powerhouse self into the forum of sports and physical activity. If you buy into the idea that an athlete's body must fit society's narrow ideal—chiseled, youthful, probably Caucasian—you are cheating the rest of us who are athletes but do not have the "right" body type. We need you in this fight to prove that we all have a place in the arena, at the starting line, on the field. For the sake of the next generation we must challenge cultural stereotypes and raise kids who see sports and health as all-inclusive.

---

**Bill Bowerman, co-founder of Nike:**
"If you have a body, you are an athlete."

---

What will it take for most people to believe that an athlete is someone proficient at sports, no matter their BMI? Seeing is believing and there is a whole tribe of women of size unleashing their inner athletes on the Internet. The images they post online have become highly influential because they help people recognize their own potential to become athletes. Plus-size yogis, runners, Olympians, and triathletes all exist and are helping to redefine what athleticism is. Here is a list of popular Instagrammers who are influencing others to embrace a new style of athleticism.

- Roz the Diva: @rozthediva
- Leah Gilbert: @leebee2321
- Jill Angie: @notyouraveragerunner
- Jessamyn Stanley: @mynameisjessamyn
- Athena Multi Sport Magazine: @athenamultisportmag
- Fat Girls' Guide to Running: @thefatgirlsguidetorunning
- Dana Falsetti: @nolatrees
- Mirna Valerio: @themirnavator
- Glitter and Lazers: @glitterandlazers
- Valerie Sagun: @biggalyoga
- Fat Girls Hiking: @fatgirlshiking
- Louise Green (me!): @Louisegreen_bigfitgirl

FOR MANY YEARS, I saw no athletes who looked like me and did not have the confidence to pursue my dreams but I finally took the leap and realized that in doing so, I could be an example myself.

---

**Whitney Way Thore, star of TLC's *My Big Fat Fabulous Life*:**
"Remember that confidence is a product of action. I rarely have the innate confidence to do something challenging; it is through my commitment to do uncomfortable things that I realize no obstacle is insurmountable, and then confidence is gained as a result. No one is born with a finite amount of confidence—it must be worked for, and it must be earned, and therefore it is an unexpected joy every time it arrives (and it will arrive over and over again, each time you force yourself outside of your comfort zone)."

---

On my journey, I discovered that I needed to replace my negative thoughts with positive ones; my "can't"s needed to turn into "can"s. This meant first acknowledging the negative thoughts and fears that were holding me back. I always thought that athletes were somehow different from me, that they had special powers that I didn't possess. I would always compare my life to theirs and focus on ways they had an advantage over me. I would make excuses, cancel my commitments to physical activity, and come up with elaborate lists of reasons why it wasn't possible for me to exercise. I now know that my fear was fueling self-sabotage.

Think about any fears you might have. Remember, fear can often show up in the form of making excuses, blaming others, being angry, and sabotaging yourself.

When I really think about what my fear was, it was ultimately fear of failure. I didn't want to put myself out there in case people found out I was a fraud and I couldn't do it. I think many of us have a fear of failure, but unless we try, we will never get to experience the victory of reaching our fitness goals. Is fear stopping you? The truth is, there *will* be failures along the way. Not every workout is fantastic or every run completed with ease, but many successful people will say that it's their failures that reap the biggest lessons and give them the strength to carry on.

Think about what obstacles lie in the way of you unleashing your inner athlete. What are you afraid of? What do you see as your barriers or excuses? I've been running my business for ten years and I think I've pretty much heard every excuse. There was traffic, I was working late, I'm sick, I've got kids, my husband needs me—it's easy to come up with reasons not to exercise. But the people I work with who really want to create change in their lives don't allow fear to smash their athletic dreams, and they create strong boundaries around their workouts to ensure their success.

Think about the barriers that hold you back and brainstorm solutions that move you closer to setting your inner athlete free. One of my barriers is that I often think I am too busy to accomplish what I set out to do. I combat this with a system I call "time management and process of elimination."

For example, one summer I had committed to four triathlons and had completed the first two, but I could feel my enthusiasm waning when it came to finishing the final two. I wanted to focus on other things, and the training was getting tiresome. As I became less committed to my goal, I found myself saying, "I am too busy," and I had to have a talk with myself. It was time for time management. I wasn't too busy. If I planned things properly and managed my time better my goals *were* possible. So, process of elimination: I reviewed a list of things that I did throughout my day and eliminated anything that wasn't getting me closer to my goal but that gave me the illusion of being "too busy." These things included watching Netflix, scrolling through social media with no real purpose, and attending certain social events. I cut them all from my agenda and then created a new training schedule, filling in the resulting holes in my day with the workouts that needed to be done. Sometimes my swims had to be done after I taught my classes in the evenings or in the early mornings before I got my son ready for school. But that's what had to happen to overcome my "busy" barrier.

My process of elimination gave me clarity and a new realization that my goals were achievable. One of my favorite tools for helping me achieve my goals is visualization, which sports psychologists now call "imaging." Our brains don't necessarily know the difference between mental visualization and actually performing the specific exercise, race, or event. Visualization or imaging helps athletes prepare for major events by tricking their brains into thinking they've already performed them.

In an article published online, the Australian Sports Commission further explains imaging:

> Mental rehearsal activates a network of neural coded programs that activate physiological responses. Therefore, imagining something means you are actually strengthening the neural pathways required for that skill and the more likely you are to reproduce it again in the future. Also by mentally practicing, you become more familiar with the actions required to perform a skill. These rehearsals make the actions more familiar or automatic.[1]

In a 2014 article titled "Olympians Use Imagery as Mental Training," the *New York Times* reported that "the practice of mentally simulating competition has become increasingly sophisticated, essential and elaborate, spilling over into realms like imagining the content of news conferences or the view from the bus window on the way to the downhill... This is, more than ever, a multisensory endeavor, which is why the term 'imaging' is now often preferred to 'visualization.'"

Whenever I prepare for a race, I imagine a successful finish. I see myself running toward the finish line. I can feel the heat coming from my face. I hear the crowds cheering louder as I approach. I can smell sweat and taste the salt on my upper lip. Once I cross the finish line I feel relief and victory. I use imaging in other areas of my life too. Mentally rehearsing makes any event feel more familiar and lessens your fear, because you've done this before and you are ready!

To be an athlete you need to start thinking like one. What will your life look like when you have unleashed your inner athlete? What does it feel like to be an athlete? Imagine the sounds, smells, and feelings associated with this vision. Try to be as specific as possible—it will make the process more effective. Perhaps you want to participate in a cycling event. Describe, to yourself, what it feels like to mount on your bike, to feel the wind on your face, and to smell the flowers in the fields as you ride past. What does it feel like to experience this freedom, and then the victory as you cross the finish line?

To seal the deal with your inner athlete, you will also need to set concrete goals. Consider everything you have ever wanted to achieve in fitness. Don't be afraid that your dream is too big; if you break that dream down into small steps, it becomes possible.

Many of us have a bucket list, and most or all of the items on it may be things we have only dreamed of doing. But that's okay. Dreaming of your bucket list is the first step to checking those items off. At first my list included running a 5K race. Later I expanded my list to include doing longer distance runs, a triathlon, and cycling in a long-distance cycling event. Now I have accomplished all of these goals and want to run a full marathon, complete a Half Ironman triathlon, and hike to the summit of Mount Kilimanjaro. My confidence and my capacity for what is possible keeps growing. I now know all these things are possible with the right planning and mindset, but there was a time when I would have laughed if someone had suggested I could achieve these goals. Even if your ideas seem foolish, I assure you they are not. Your dreams are something to be taken seriously, and they are absolutely doable. Whatever barriers you see in the way are surmountable. But to get past those barriers, you must first change your mindset and believe that it is possible to overcome them.

HERE IS MY step-by-step story, including the past, the moment of transition, and the present, showing how I made the change from nonbeliever to believer and from dreamer to athlete. I had to knock down barriers, change my behaviors, and conquer my fear to get from where I was then to today.

THEN: Fitness wasn't a priority. Other things got in the way, including parties, socializing, and just sitting on the couch. Fitness wasn't important to the people I spent time with either.

TRANSITION: I slowly started making fitness a larger part of my life one commitment and event at a time. I signed up for my first running clinic and made some new friends there with a similar interest in running. After that I felt confident enough to sign up for my first 5K run. With each success, my confidence increased. It became easier to carve out time for fitness as I experienced the physical and emotional benefits of being active. With my newfound zest for life I started to believe in myself, something I didn't have much experience with in the past. I was fortunate to find a community of runners who became my peer network. By surrounding myself with others who believed in the value of fitness and made it a priority in their lives, I was continually inspired.

NOW: Fitness is a top priority in my life. I make a plan for each year that includes my fitness goals, and add all my workouts to my calendar. I look at each goal and to support them I find training plans either for free from the Internet or by purchasing a plan from an online coaching company. I incorporate these plans into my calendar and then work my social events around them as opposed to working my plans around my socializing; putting fitness second wasn't very successful in the past. Each workout supports the next, and I know that my efforts will be rewarded because I've put a solid plan in place.

THEN: I didn't have the self-confidence to step outside of my comfort zone, so I played it safe and stuck to my usual routines. I hung out with the same friends, we went to the same places for drinks, and then I'd go home and sit on the couch dreaming of another life. I didn't want to throw my life off-course. That did nothing to help me achieve my athletic dreams. True wins are rarely accomplished by always staying inside your comfort zone.

TRANSITION: I got to a place where I knew that if I wanted to follow my dreams, fear (and conquering it) would be part of my life. As I completed events and achieved goals, I realized that pushing against fear for my own betterment is healthy. My success gave me the motivation I needed to keep going. It is in action that we build confidence to persevere.

NOW: I understand that stepping out of my comfort zone and experiencing fear is part of the process of growth. I have faced fear so many times now that it feels normal. My accomplishments have shown me that I will not combust or die if I do something that I fear. Fear is just energy, excitement about the unknown, and I no longer see it as something to avoid

THEN: I didn't know where to go or what to do. I viewed

many fitness activities as "not for me." This came from my fear that I wasn't capable of particular activities or wasn't welcome in that world. I feared what people thought and didn't want to look foolish if I couldn't perform. I craved acceptance.

TRANSITION: I decided that pursuing fitness was about me and not about anyone else. What others thought of me was not my concern and was no reflection on my own self-worth. I needed to show up—to classes, to a run, to just be present—for me. Perhaps this is the stage you are at right now? If so, ease into your new routine. I started with one goal and took my physical transformation one step at a time. Showing up for yourself is the first step in figuring it all out.

NOW: I don't let other people's judgments deter me from pursuing my dreams. I really don't care what people think of me because now I don't need others' approval to elevate my sense of self-worth. My self-worth now comes from within. I've also come to realize that most athletic communities are very supportive and welcoming. Many people are happy to welcome newcomers, no matter who they are or what their size is, to their sport or activity, and to help them learn and feel more comfortable.

THEN: I didn't have people in my life who participated in fitness or sports. The people around me didn't view health or fitness as a priority.

TRANSITION: As I slowly engaged more regularly in fitness activities, I began to attract people into my life who were also interested in fitness and athletics. As my interest in fitness grew, I started reading books and articles about fitness, buying new gear, and talking with like-minded people. My new tribe started to grow, and I strengthened friendships with people whose priorities were fitness rather than drinking on a Friday night into the early hours. This helped me shift my own priorities and create a new lifestyle.

NOW: The people in my life now are goal-oriented and active. They too believe that life is limitless, and they help me find this positive energy within myself. Their enthusiasm when we gather to enjoy our favorite sports is infectious, and their own commitment—to their activities and to supporting me—inspires me to keep going.

THEN: I never allowed myself to achieve my goals. Once I got close to making exercise a consistent part of my life, I'd often back away and sabotage my efforts. Things would get hard, and being fit was uncharted territory out of my comfort zone. I would eventually start making excuses for why the exercise wasn't going to work, and I would revert to my usual activities—drinking wine and watching television.

TRANSITION: I started to recognize my self-sabotage, which was usually a result of my fear. I would have a chat with myself to overcome the urge to back out of an activity, overriding my negative thoughts with positive comments such as "You deserve this. This is what you want. You signed up for this; don't give up!" I had to teach myself to feel worthy enough to reach my goals.

NOW: I recognize self-sabotage immediately, including the subtle ways I try to avoid a workout. I still do it today; I'll tell myself I'm too tired, or my family needs me.

Fear is the biggest cause of lost dreams. If we can recognize it and respect it as part of the process, it becomes normal and surmountable. I recognize that each workout is integral to my success. Not showing up is no longer an option, and every excuse I've ever come up with is familiar to me. I now know the reasons behind them, so they no longer work!

As the saying goes, "Rome wasn't built in a day." With every accomplishment, my goals increase ever-so-slightly. I tell myself, "Well, if I can run three minutes without stopping, I can probably run five minutes." My accomplishments just keep building and expanding. I have realized that—within reason—if I can dream it, plan for it, and put in the training time, then the sky is the limit. If I allow myself to think it, then it is possible. This is the Big Fit Girl mindset.

## Nine Habits of Highly Successful Athletes

OVER THE YEARS I have watched athletes I admire and tried to emulate the behavior that I believe led to their success. Wonderful things resulted. My dedication to a fit life expanded, and I continued to make my athletic dreams reality. Here are some of the habits I observed in these athletes:

1. They think positively and visualize success in their lives.
2. They set goals, both short-term and long-term, and create solid action plans to support their goals.
3. They follow structured training plans or add their workouts to a calendar. Each workout or training session is part of a bigger picture.
4. They keep records or logs to track their progress. Measurement is important, though I recognize it is not for everyone. Keep an open mind: keeping track of your progress allows you to see how far you have come. This is a great motivator when self-sabotage comes into play.
5. They work out even when they don't want to, because they know they will feel great afterward and be happy they did so. Not every workout is something you will gleefully want to do, but your mindset quickly changes as endorphins are released. These athletes also understand that every workout is part of the big picture and there are seldom shortcuts.
6. They practice self-discipline and avoid the temptations of life if these get in the way of their goals (staying out too late, drinking too much, sleeping in).

7. They are willing to do whatever it takes to achieve their goals. They will get up early, run in the rain, or train before a social event (instead of skipping the training) if they have to.

8. They have self-compassion. Not all workouts will be great, but successful athletes learn from their not-so-good workouts and their mistakes and see shortcomings as opportunities to improve. Everyone has a bad workout sometimes. Highly successful athletes know this and show up anyway.

9. They are social beings, and most train with groups, coaches, or teams at least some of the time. They value the opportunity to learn from fellow athletes, as well as to push themselves with friendly competitors.

PART OF BEING a Big Fit Girl is thinking like an athlete. Adopt some of these nine habits for a step in the right direction. They will help you to consistently put in the hard work it takes to achieve goals. Keep this list in mind as you create a plan for how you will unleash your inner athlete!

## What Activities Work Best for Plus-Size Women?

YOU ARE LIMITED only by your own fear. There is no "right" activity for a plus-size woman, just as there is no "right" activity for someone with a smaller body who is new to fitness. You may have heard people suggest you try these typical activities: water aerobics, swimming, yoga, or walking. These activities are often recommended because they are seen as gentler and more manageable for bigger bodies. After hitting the pool to swim some laps, I am not sure I agree that swimming is gentle! And there are some pretty tough water aerobics and yoga classes out there. If you go at your own pace, the sky is the limit.

What activity is right for you? Start with what you enjoy, not what you or others think you are capable of. Try a few different activities to see what feels the best. With the right training, a community of support, and your own determination, you can achieve anything. Rather than give you a list of exercises made for larger bodies, I turned to my favorite athletes (they happen to be plus-size) to share their favorite fitness activities. Which one speaks to you? What do you feel inspired to try?

## Yoga

### KRYSTAL THOMPSON, OWNER OF THE LUSCIOUS LIFE

Early forms of yoga were developed by the Indus-Sarasvati civilization in Northern India over 5,000 years ago. Yoga is practiced every day, by millions of people, all around the world. Although modern-day yoga can appear intimidating, people of all shapes and sizes are busting out their warrior pose. I met yoga teacher Krystal Thompson at the Body Love Conference in Tucson, Arizona. Her passion for yoga inspired me to ask her more. Here is her story:

> I started my yoga practice in 1997. Yoga felt like a safer form of moving my bigger body in public than something like running or joining another sport. I had very self-limiting beliefs about my body and what it could do back then. Yoga felt easier for me to access because I had a background in dance that had developed my body awareness and flexibility.
>
> Through my regular and disciplined yoga practice I have discovered that I am more than my body and I am definitely more than the way my body looks. My worth and my value are more than a number on a scale. My physical ability and athleticism are more than the size of my body. It was a slow and subtle process, but the power of yoga brought me to this place.

Asana taught me about strength I didn't know I had. It taught me about breathing through challenge. It taught me about the incredible ability and power of my body that has nothing to do with what anyone else thinks. It is through my dedication to yoga, and to becoming a yoga teacher, that I began to love my body and love my life.

Yoga offers endless health benefits—improved balance, muscular strength, flexibility, and posture—and it can be a great tool for stress management.

You can find yoga in most towns and cities; it is just a matter of locating a studio where you feel comfortable. There are many yoga programs available online if starting in your home feels right. I recommend the Cody Fitness app (codyapp.com) for downloading yoga programs for people of all shapes and sizes.

## Running

**SHANNON SVINGEN-JONES, FOUNDER AND EDITOR-IN-CHIEF AT *FABUPLUS MAGAZINE***

Shannon and I have a lot in common: we both love running, and running built our confidence to pursue our larger athletic dreams. Shannon is now editor-in-chief at her magazine *FabUplus*, which shows plus-size women that a healthy and fit lifestyle is possible. Here is what she has to say:

I never would have imagined myself as a runner, never in a million years. As a plus-size woman, I always felt that my body wasn't built for it. I had also heard many tales about running—"runners have bad knees"; "runners get so many injuries"—so I just stayed away. It wasn't until a good friend of mine who had recently taken up running challenged me to a 10K race—she knew me oh-too-well, as I never turn down a challenge. I began training, I downloaded a learn-to-run schedule online, and off I went. Going in, I was fully prepared to walk the entire race, but after following the training schedule, I realized that I could do it. I could actually run, and I loved it.

I ended up doing that first race without stopping once, and this race led me to more, and one more, and one more. When you train slowly and safely, it can be for any body. Running is the new love of my life. It works great for me because it's free, you can do it in groups or by yourself, and at any time of the day.

Most cities and towns have running programs affiliated with a sporting goods store. If you find that your area doesn't offer a running program, there are plenty online that you can download.

## Walking

### MICHELLE SWEET, MARATHON WALKER AND ATHLETE

Michelle is one of my clients, and her transformation has been incredible to watch. I love hearing the stories of people who have found a love for exercise and who have transformed from fitness-loather to fitness-lover. These transformations confirm that deep within all of us there *is* an athlete, perhaps one that had been waiting for the right fitness fit. If you can unearth your inner athlete by participating in something you truly love, then exercise will be your friend for life. Here's Michelle's story:

I have never been what I would consider an athletic person. For me and my larger frame, physical activity was a chore, and I was embarrassed to participate. I was thrilled when I was able to drop Physical Education at the start of grade 11, as it was no longer a mandatory subject. I began to find my inner athlete begrudgingly a couple of years ago, at the age of forty-three, when I met my current doctor, who insisted that I get a minimum of thirty minutes of activity per day. My primary preference was walking, and I was reasonably disciplined, maybe not hitting my thirty minutes every day, but most.

However, recently a friend of mine posted something on Facebook: "A walk a day and a photo along the way," with a picture of herself and a picture of some scenery from her walk. I asked her if I could copy her. She gave her blessing and I started my "Walk a day and a pic along the way" journey. Best decision ever! Not only did it keep me accountable, but it sparked a passion inside of me for fitness. Now I have signed up to walk my very first marathon, in Honolulu!

My whole life is changing weekly. My physical ability and skills are improving each and every day. I am getting healthier and happier one step at a time. This is the new me, and I wouldn't change a thing!

Walking is so accessible—perhaps walking is your way to athleticism?

Like running programs, walking programs can be found in most cities or towns. If you find that your area doesn't offer one, download a walking program from the Internet and get started.

## Triathlon

### LEAH GILBERT, TRIATHLETE AND FOUNDER OF BODY POSITIVE ATHLETES

Leah is one of the women who influenced me to get into triathlons. Seeing her participate and coach others showed me I could do it too. Leah strongly advocates that all bodies can join in the sport of triathlon. Triathlon is my new favorite sport. It allows me to have variety in training over the three disciplines. If you get bored easily like me, this is a great way to stay on your toes! If you are willing to put in the time and training, triathlon might be for you. Here's Leah's story:

> I had always secretly dreamed of doing a triathlon but had never gone through the training or tried to complete one, because I just didn't think I would ever be able to do it.
>
> After I started running in 2013 and got my distance up, I purchased a bike in order to do some cross-training. As my bike distance increased, I realized I was doing the distances of some smaller triathlons. All I had to do was put all these activities together. I started researching triathlon training approaches, and the rest is history.
>
> Triathlon has allowed me to unleash my inner athlete, because you can't train for a triathlon and *not* be an athlete. Training for this sport requires you to develop fitness, speed, and skills across three disciplines, so to even sustain training you must be in an athletic headspace. Quite often the athletic lifestyle is just a side effect of getting all your training done!
>
> Triathlon has finally given me the platform to unleash the disciplined, determined athlete I knew I always had deep within me.

Many cities and towns will offer triathlon clubs that offer group training and camaraderie. However, some are good for beginners and some are not. It's a good idea to reach out to them and get a feel for the group by being honest about your starting position. If the club can't accommodate you they will likely know who can. Alternatively, you can seek out online coaching or download triathlon training plans, but whenever possible, train with a group or training partner for the most success.

## Cycling

### NATALIE DZANY, LONG-DISTANCE CYCLIST

I first read about Natalie in an article she wrote about plus-size clothing; I later looked her up and we connected. We became fast Internet friends and realized we have a lot in common. Natalie is an athlete and has participated in many long-distance cycling events. Cycling isn't all about distance, but Natalie demonstrates that both short and long distances are possible for all bodies. Here is Natalie's story:

> My love for cycling started when I was a kid, but it was only a few years ago that I started signing up for cycling challenges. I started with some 25K rides, and then I biked a 100K challenge. Now I do several cycling events a year. I was able to build my distance by staying consistent, and if cycling interests you, you can too. I also use my bicycle as a means of transportation, and I ride about 25K daily to and from work. Through these events, and by using my bike to get around, I have definitely unleashed my inner athlete! For me, cycling equals freedom. It's my bicycle, nature, and me, and I go as far as my legs will take me. I'm a long-distance cyclist, so there are no time trials or milestones. The longer the ride, the stronger I feel.
>
> Every kilometer I ride makes me realize how strong my legs are, and I'm thankful each and every time. It's not about how I look; it's about how I feel, and I feel fabulous!
>
> Cycling is a great choice of activity because it is fairly accessible, it's free (once you have a bike), and it offers a great cardiovascular workout without high impact.

Once you have a bike cycling is a very accessible sport. Most urban centers are well planned with cycling routes and many cities offer green spaces with park paths. There's also the option to do indoor cycling, which may appeal if you live in a climate where it's not possible to cycle in the winter. Community centers often run spin classes and most cities boast indoor cycling centers.

## Weight Training / CrossFit

### SYLVIA KLOBUCAR, CROSSFIT COMPETITOR

Sylvia—I call her "Sylv"—is another incredible athlete I met in the online community of plus-size athletes. I originally found Sylv through the community Body Positive Athletes and was intrigued by her journey to the CrossFit games. The images of her lifting heavy weights were incredibly powerful. Here is Sylv's story:

> I originally took up CrossFit to increase my strength training to help me out in the other sports I partake in. It didn't take long to smash all my misconceptions about the sport and about plus-size CrossFitters.
>
> CrossFit introduces Olympic weight lifting to their routines, but you're not lifting Olympic-level weights from the start. In fact, you need to do the fundamental sessions, learning correct lifting and movement techniques, before you lift anything heavier than a plastic pipe. Safety and injury prevention are important in CrossFit.
>
> If you're worried about your fitness level or aggravating pre-existing injuries, don't be. The coaches at CrossFit will scale the workout to your level. Every workout is different but covers cardio and strength training, so there's no shortage of variety. While you may compete against yourself in CrossFit, you end up becoming part of a community which doubles as a cheer squad cheering on other members when they achieve a goal.

If you want a sport where you can progress at your own pace, unleash your inner athlete, and really learn what your body and mind are capable of, then CrossFit may just be for you!

There are more than 13,000 CrossFit gyms around the world, and more than half of them are in North America. Regular weight training can be found at any gym. Personal trainers can coach individuals in weight training with free weights and machines; however, Olympic weight training and power lifting is fairly specialized. Lifts such as the "snatch" and "clean and jerk" require experienced coaching; for your safety, I recommend making sure the trainer you choose is well-versed in technique.

## Hiking

**EDITH BERNIER, TRAVEL BLOGGER & AUTHOR**

Edith is a fellow Canadian plus-size fitness enthusiast who focuses on the joys of hiking and backpacking at every size. I was intrigued to follow Edith because she offers specialized information about plus-size backpacking in her book, *The Ultimate Guide to Plus-Size Backpacking.* Here is Edith's story:

> I like to explore and take photographs when I travel, and hiking allowed me to reach more remote areas. From Mayan ruins in the heart of the jungle to solidified lava fields, hiking has helped me to discover harder-to-reach gems of our world and to unleash my inner athlete.
>
> What is great about hiking is how accessible it is. You can do it anytime, anywhere, almost all year long, and all you need is a good pair of shoes (and a hiking stick in rougher terrain). You can do it in a group or alone. Because it is a low-impact

sport with a minimal risk of injury, you can recover in a day or two from even the toughest hike.

To push your limits, you can either increase your pace or the level of difficulty of the path. Being at the bottom of a steep trail may really make you doubt your capacity to make it to the top, though going back is not always an option, especially when in a group. This kind of situation can push you to do something you never thought possible. I have overestimated myself occasionally, but I admit it's a great way to stay motivated, as it makes me want to train harder to be able to go farther, higher, and faster.

If you live in the right place, hiking is an accessible activity that offers beauty and freedom. Nature is a fabulous place to connect with yourself and clear your mind. Maybe hiking is your thing?

## Dance

**WHITNEY WAY THORE, DANCER AND STAR OF TLC'S *MY BIG FAT FABULOUS LIFE***

Whitney became famous for her YouTube video titled "A Fat Girl Dancing," which has been viewed more than two million times. She is a lifelong dancer experienced in ballet, tap, jazz, and hip-hop. She obtained her Zumba teaching license in 2011 and now teaches a class called "Big Girl Dance," which provides a safe space for people of every ability, gender, and race to experience the excitement and joy of dance; she also produced a DVD series called "Werk with Whitney." Here is Whitney's story:

Dance comes naturally to me; it was the first physical activity I allowed my fat body to do ten years after I first began to gain a significant amount of weight. I felt safe while I was dancing. I didn't need any special equipment or a partner—just music and the ability to let go. Once I realized that fat girls could indeed dance, I decided to see what else I could do and was delighted to find joy again at the gym, in sports, and in recreational exercise.

The benefits of dance are endless for everyone, but plus-size women especially. Dance includes intuitive movement, so each woman may begin to move her body in the ways that feel most natural to her—there's no wrong way to do it! It's also a great social skill, which may help women feel more confident about going to clubs or events where dancing is involved. I love dance because it allows limitless expression. From tap to twerking, there is something for everyone. Dance is an integral part of cultures all around the world because it connects your heart to your body and people to each other.

A wide range of dance classes is offered through most community centers and dance companies, and many offer programming for new or returning dancers. Dance is a great way to express yourself and to lose yourself in exercise!

## Boxing

ONE OF MY favorite fitness specialties is boxing. I've been boxing and coaching women in the sport for many years and within my classes, it is by far the component that elicits the most power, effort, and sweat. From what I have witnessed, I've concluded that women love to hit things! In addition to boosting strength and cardiovascular fitness, boxing improves coordination, power, and reaction times so that you are ready for anything life throws at you.

It is also a great way to release stress, engage in a wicked cardiovascular session, and learn self-defense skills. One of the reasons I choose to train women through boxing is because it offers a killer interval-style cardio without impact on knees, hips, or ankles. Because you have to learn and keep up with specific combos, it also offers great opportunity for mental fitness. My ladies love boxing! Maybe boxing is for you too?

Boxing training is performed by hitting pads or targets or a punching bag, not actual opponents in a ring, so it's safe, fun, and challenging.

Some cities and towns offer women-specific boxing programs, but if they don't exist you can look for gyms or boxing clubs that offer co-ed boxing.

## Swimming

SWIMMING IS ONE of my favorite forms of exercise. About two years ago I started participating in triathlons. Of course, this meant I had to swim! For me, this was the scariest part of doing a triathlon. I'd never swum lengths before, so I was starting from scratch. At first I practiced on my own but started to realize my stroke technique needed improving and was holding me back. I joined a swim course, which included three hours of in-class instruction on swim technique and two hours of in-pool teaching. The instructor filmed us swimming and then we discussed ways to improve our form. From there I enrolled in a regular adult swimming program that focused on stroke technique for the four main strokes: front crawl, breaststroke, backstroke, and butterfly. I put a lot into learning how to swim with good technique because in triathlon, swimming with efficiency is an integral part of a successful race. I was amazed at how much I loved it, and today, it's one of my favorite parts of triathlon.

What I love about swimming is that you can build strength fairly quickly. Swimming lengths can be challenging but also encouraging; there are all kinds of people at the pool, and different lanes for swimmers of different speeds, so you can go at your own pace. Swimming builds muscles with the resistance from the water but doesn't negatively affect your joints. This means swimming is a challenging workout that is also safe. I find I also get a killer cardiovascular workout, while building strength—all from one great session. There's also something calming about being in the water—it feels good for the soul.

Swimming lessons are offered by most community centers as well as by private clubs. I did my first swim program through a company that specialized in triathlon swimming, but I found my adult lessons at the local rec center. If you are interested in perfecting your stroke check out what your community offers. There are generally swimming programs for all levels. I've progressed to open water swimming lessons, wetsuit and all!

THESE ACTIVITIES ARE just the tip of the iceberg: there's also tennis, mud racing, pole dancing for fitness, Nordic walking, snowshoeing, and so much more. Take some time to think about what might work for you. When you read the stories of athletes in the previous pages, which one piqued your interest the most? Do some research and see what's available in your community. Don't worry about what the fitness magazines say—there's more to fitness than running or lunging with weights in the gym. Create your own fitness fit. You have the power to become a Big Fit Girl in your own way.

---

**Marcy Cruz, lifestyle blogger and blog editor at *PLUS Model Magazine*:**
"I love to walk. The actual walking part is easy for me. The hardest part is getting out of bed and out of the house. But once I am out of the house, I feel like a free bird. My feet have taken me to so many wonderful places. They have served me so well in life. So why not use them to walk and get healthy while seeing the world at the same time?"

---

FIND SOMETHING THAT works for you and your body, as well as something you can sustain and make an enjoyable part of your life. Once you have identified and overcome the obstacles standing in your way and built your confidence by taking action, you will be limitless.

You are an athlete. Say it out loud: "I am an athlete." This is your new daily mantra! Now it is time to live it.

# THREE

# Creating Your Master Team

N O ONE WHO has achieved greatness has done it alone. My journey has shown me that you need supportive people around you. Your people are the difference between success and failure; they help you make it, stick with it, and enjoy the journey.

I have been fortunate: the right people have lifted me up, encouraged me, and shown me through their own example what is possible. They are my trainers, tribes, and teams, and they have pushed me to achieve success.

I have also encountered the wrong people. I think we all have. I want to tell you a story about one such meeting that profoundly shaped me. My hope is that this story will help you shape your team with the right people.

## Doctor Brown Town

IT'S A TYPICAL scenario: the first time you meet a doctor, you arrive right on time, only to be told to sit in a sterile brown and beige room, where you wait and wait and wait. The edge of your irritation softens when it is finally your turn—as it was mine after more than twenty minutes.

Rushed and disheveled, a man in his late fifties finally strode into the tiny examination room where I sat. Dressed entirely in taupe and brown, he matched the office decor. He barely looked at me before sitting down at a computer and typing. When he finally glanced over at me, without a word of introduction, he barked: "How much do you weigh?"

I felt a lump forming in my throat because I knew this visit was heading in a negative direction. "Two hundred and twenty pounds," I said.

"Height," he demanded.

He entered the number into the computer, then turned to look down at me through his wire-rimmed bifocal glasses. He sighed. "That's a BMI of 35." And, without softening the blow, "Your health is at risk."

He didn't ask me about my physical activity—I was running 30K a week. He didn't remark on my perfect health—below average blood pressure, balanced cholesterol, and optimal blood sugar. He didn't even ask why I had come to see him.

Right then and there I knew I'd never come back to Dr. Brown Town. He simply couldn't be a part of my master team. I stood up and walked out. If you ever have a similar experience—if you encounter someone who wants to judge and label, and not understand, support, and encourage—I hope you stand up and walk out too.

We need our support team to treat us as human beings and individuals, not as a series of calculations that may or may not be accurate (Body Mass Index, or BMI, is a particularly archaic measurement that was devised in the 1800s and better applied to population studies rather than individual assessments). My first running coach, Chris, in contrast to Dr. Brown Town, never mentioned weight, weight loss, BMI, or cultural stereotypes.

Had she not been accepting of size diversity, would I have ever started running? If Dr. Brown Town had been my only encounter with health professionals, would I have simply given up on my athletic dreams?

Sitting in my car after my doctor's appointment, I was filled with anger and disappointment. I had been judged, without a second thought, because of my appearance.

This experience was in stark contrast with my encounters with people who did not judge my capabilities and health by my size; in those cases I felt encouraged to keep working toward my goals. I call this a "weight-neutral" approach, which simply means that people don't make any assumptions about your health or fitness based on your appearance.

HEALTH AT EVERY SIZE is a prime example of a movement taking a weight-neutral approach. HAES supports people in adopting healthy habits for the sake of well-being rather than weight control. It aims to remove the discrimination associated with larger bodies and to improve the standard of living for people who are fat. HAES believes that traditional restrictive dieting is not always healthful and that it does not always result in sustained weight loss. It proposes that health is a result of behaviors that are independent of body weight and that societal obsession with thinness does not allow for diversity in acceptable body shapes. HAES has recently gained popularity as an alternative to weight loss. Clearly Dr. Brown Town hadn't gotten the memo.

I've noted that I'm the most motivated when I address change from a weight-neutral perspective. I want this to be your reality too.

Weight neutrality starts by surrounding yourself with people who are open to the idea that health and fitness are possible at different sizes. Through their support, these people show they do not believe there are limits to your achievements. You need a supportive environment in order to achieve long-term success: a study by Leah Gilbert's Body Positive Athletes, a company in Australia, found that 85 percent of respondents reported that a body-positive training environment was extremely important to their long-term participation in physical activity. A body-positive training environment is one that is judgment-free, is focused on fitness, and actively discourages dieting. Essentially, it embodies the HAES ethos.

How can you find environments that are supportive and encouraging? I've identified three groups that have helped me get where I am today, and depending on your budget and interest in being social while exercising, you can build similar support groups for your own journey. You need a trainer, a tribe, and a team.

## The Trainer

THE TRAINER OR coach is your mentor and guide to your physical fitness efforts. As a mentor who has worked with thousands of women, I know this is an intimate relationship. I have been privy to deeply personal information that allows me to better understand a person's life and what has brought that person to me. Because this is a highly personal relationship, it is important that you choose the right trainer.

You should be able to find a good trainer through the Internet. Search for keywords and phrases such as: "body-positive fitness," "weight neutral," "HAES trainers," "size friendly," "plus-size fitness," or "fitness for all levels."

You are the CEO of your body, and like any CEO, you have the power to allow people into your space or to dismiss them if they're not doing a good job. All good CEOs carefully interview candidates for a position to ensure that they fit the culture and have the experience and knowledge to handle the job. I often find that those who have not had good experiences with health and fitness do not properly vet people when they are establishing their support systems. After managing phone and email inquiries for many years, I have found that people frequently begin by apologizing for their weight or health and fitness and put the trainers and health professionals in the power position. They also tend to describe their current state of fitness as far worse than it actually is, establishing a hierarchy between themselves and the trainer.

Keep your power like a CEO would. You need to interview every member of your master team. I can't stress this enough. Interview people as if the success of your hopes and dreams depends on it—because it does.

Before you conduct an interview, you must first know what is important to you. Each of us needs different qualities in a trainer. You might prefer a female trainer, or you may want someone who is close to your age; you may want a gentle trainer, or someone more challenging. The main thing to figure out when you interview someone is whether or not that person ticks your boxes, whatever they might be. There isn't just one version of success. What do you need from a trainer? Here is my list of requirements for trainers.

1. They should be accredited.
2. They should have personal experience in the activity or the goals I want to pursue—in my current case, to compete in a triathlon.
3. They must be reliable and professional at all times. This means that they must be punctual and focus their full attention on me. For example, I once had a trainer who would put me on a cardio machine and then go sit in her office texting on her phone. I felt insignificant, and she had to go.

4. They should be friendly but have high expectations of me and push me beyond what I would do myself.
5. They must understand that my goals do not include weight loss as the focus; rather, they must focus on creating activities that challenge my fitness achievements. I am open to nutritional advice for performance and good health but not restrictive plans for losing weight.

Take a moment to think about what is important to you in a trainer. What qualities do you want and not want? Once you have identified your list of wants, it becomes easier to craft a set of interview questions that allow you to discover the right person.

I recommend prefacing your interview by saying something like this: "My health and fitness is important to me, and working with the right people is paramount to my success. Are you open to some questions to explore how we might work together?"

If the response is anything other than yes, that is a major red flag and this trainer should not even get a tryout for the team. Most trainers are happy to talk it through to see if the two of you make a good fit.

**QUESTIONS TO ASK A TRAINER:**
- Do you believe that healthy and fit bodies come in a range of shapes and sizes?
- If the gym advertises all-inclusive fitness: What is your all-inclusive training approach? What makes it all-inclusive and how will my specific needs be met?
- What's your approach to healthy nutrition?
- What is your experience working with the plus-size demographic?
- Can you give me some examples of exercises I might perform?

- In one sentence, describe your training style.
- Have you ever been fat?
- Do you have any testimonials or references from other clients? If so, may I contact them?
- What is the training environment like? Can I come and see the facility or space before I commit?

These are just some examples of questions to ask to make sure there is a right fit before you've signed contracts, paid a lot of money, and locked yourself in.

Don't underestimate the importance of a good training environment. You want to feel comfortable in the space where you work out. I once hired a trainer at a gym that had been converted from an old health club. The weight area was inside a converted racquetball court and it was dark and dingy with no natural light. What's more, the cardio machines upstairs looked down on the training area. The gym was a popular choice for body-building guys who liked to grunt loudly while they worked out. I found myself training in a gloomy gym, surrounded by bulky grunting men, while thirty people stared down at me from the treadmills above. At three months postpartum, I was at my heaviest and feeling very self-conscious. Had I viewed the training setup before signing on the dotted line, I would have gone elsewhere.

Most of the questions on my list are ones I have posed to trainers in the past, and most of those trainers have been happy to answer. I've also had similar questions asked of me many, many times. I often answer the questions before they are even asked because I know from experience what a potential client often wants to know. But if a trainer doesn't offer the information up front, asking questions will give you a better idea if they are a right fit and helps to establish a level of trust. I also offer a complimentary session so that people can try before they buy.

This gesture further signifies that I am committed to making this a win/win relationship before any money changes hands. Many fitness establishments will allow a complimentary trial or facility tour, so always ask if there's an opportunity to "try before you buy."

Asking the right questions will expose a trainer's belief system and training philosophy. You want to be sure you are compatible with his or her vision of wellness and that the trainer sees things the way you do.

You may be saying to yourself: "Okay, but I'm new at this. How do I know what the trainer's answers really mean?" Here are answers that should raise red flags:

- I believe in high-intensity interval training and clean eating plans of 1200 calories to get your body trimmed down for optimum health.
- I think that excess weight is unhealthy: calories in, calories out.
- No, I've never been heavy; I work out eight times a week to avoid it.
- Never heard of health at every size, but c'mon, fat people can't be healthy.
- Let's get you beach body ready!

You might be thinking, "A trainer wouldn't really say those things!" I have found that the fitness industry—the industry I am so passionate about—can be very unaccepting of diverse views about health and fitness. There are some really invested trainers, but due diligence is a must.

Here are some answers that sound more promising:

- Yes, I struggled with my weight as a child; it's been really challenging, but I figured out what works for me.

- I do believe that a range of body sizes can be fit and healthy; in fact, my weight has fluctuated and some of my biggest fitness achievements have been at my heavier weights.
- I've never been heavy but I do everything possible to understand how I can best serve my clients' needs at all sizes.
- I support a weight neutral approach and help my clients achieve an active lifestyle to accompany that style.
- Healthy nutrition means eating healthy food and fueling your body to perform like an athlete but also enjoying some treats.

ANDREA GUZZO IS a personal trainer and boot camp owner who specializes in training plus-size women. When new clients call, Andrea knows if they are apprehensive about becoming active and she tries to address their fears and concerns immediately. She explains that her classes are inclusive and she teaches both women who have been coming for years and those who are new. She assures people that she can tailor exercises to meet the physical needs of each individual. With many years of experience working with plus-size women, Andrea can modify exercises quickly to suit the needs of her clients no matter what their level. Her fitness classes foster a supportive atmosphere and her clients encourage each other in class. Andrea has developed a welcoming space for people to sweat, and in the process, created a supportive community.

With personal training clients, Andrea listens carefully to fully understand their goals. For example, her client Vicky wanted to add additional activity hours to her week. Andrea tries to get a good idea of what is realistic for each client, and she asked Vicky if she was willing to track her workouts in a journal. At first Vicky resisted Andrea's suggestion, so they made a deal. Andrea said she would journal too, and then they could meet for coffee, compare notes, and offer each other advice on improvement. Andrea joining Vicky in her homework created a feeling of teamwork, and as a result Vicky knew they were accountable to each other. Andrea proposed that Vicky increase her fitness by adding two additional walks to her weekly activity, and then she reviewed all the homework at their next meeting. From there they made further plans and adjustments as needed. Weekly reviews are a big part of Andrea's routine: if her clients don't meet their homework requirements, they study their journals together and figure out where the process failed and create solutions for the next week.

Andrea is a deeply invested trainer and did everything right with Vicky. She created trust with Vicky by hearing her out and fully understanding what her goals were. She didn't project her own goals onto Vicky. Meeting with Vicky made her accountable and brought Vicky closer to her goals.

HERE ARE SOME of the qualities of a good trainer:

- Good trainers are invested in your goals. They take the time to hear what you would like to achieve. They do not project their own goals onto you.
- They never squash your big goals but instead set up small steps to help you reach these milestones in due time. A good trainer will love that you have big goals and will be excited to tackle them with you.
- They share your values of health and wellness.
- They will not give you high-intensity exercises or drills that reflect their own workouts or feed their own ego while risking client injury or burnout.
- They are committed to making exercise fun and attainable for you.
- They focus on making every session feel like you've achieved great success as you walk out the door.

- They adapt and modify to ensure your safety and success.
- They work with your fitness level and slowly increase intensity levels as time goes on.
- They understand that exercises feel different to people who are bigger and take that into consideration when planning programs and classes.
- They are trained to read body language, facial cues, and other nonverbal communication, such as levels of perspiration or breathing, to determine whether the level of intensity, or Rate of Perceived Exertion (RPE), is appropriate.
- And finally, they know their audience and use appropriate language when explaining exercises and motivating their clients. Trainers should never use body-shaming tactics to motivate a client. For example, they shouldn't say, "Okay, ladies, summer's coming. There is not much time to get bikini ready, so let's work hard!" Instead, they could say: "You are all amazing athletes. Let's keep giving it everything we've got. You're unstoppable!"

## The Tribe

YOUR TRIBE, ALSO known as your community of fellow exercisers, is crucial to unleashing your Big Fit Girl.

Jen is one of the longest-term clients of the training program I own. She has been coming to our program for over five years, and she attributes her commitment to both our supportive trainers and her tribe:

I have always been fortunate to have a supportive group of friends, but when I first started at boot camp it was so frightening to me because it was a new environment. I was in fear of failure and of judgment. After the first class, those feelings disappeared. I was accepted so easily, and nobody judged me. It helped me realize I could do this, and as time went by, it pushed me to take on different challenges. Knowing that I wasn't alone in my initial feelings of fear helped too. To have these women truly understand what goes on when you live in a larger body and exercise, and to have a cohesive tribe doing it together, only fuels me to do more. In the past, people were shocked that I was so active but now I have people asking for my advice. People tell me I have inspired them to engage in fitness, and it proves that I am making a difference, one mind at time.

Fitness friends are what make fitness stick. Your tribe will support your goals, and they will notice when you're not at your session. The people in your tribe will become your accountability partners, helping to ensure that you never turn your back on your goals. They will be there for you when times are tough, when you don't feel like showing up, and through setbacks like injury and illness. This is a very special bond that is fostered over time.

SHARON IS A plus-size athlete who has finally found her tribe. Not surprisingly, she has now also reached new levels of fitness. She didn't feel comfortable going to a conventional gym to exercise. She researched a number of places but felt too intimidated by the ultra-buff-looking clientele. One day she read about a fitness company that focused on plus-size people. It became her fitness haunt.

It was a highly supportive environment where everyone was at different fitness levels, but no one judged you or expected you to perform at a set level. The community supported me, and I learned that a person's potential to succeed and exceed what they think they are capable of doing is much higher when they are part of a supportive and inclusive community. The key is seeing people around you of all different shapes and sizes, some smaller and some bigger. Everybody is trying their best and supporting each other. No one is judging you based on how firm your abs are or what your butt looks like.

Sometimes your tribe is just one other person, and finding the right person is really important. It can be difficult to find the right match and many of us have failed on our first attempt. I've had a couple of training partners that just couldn't follow through or who had a negative mindset during training, and the negativity wore me down. You can't be positive one hundred percent of the time when you're feeling especially challenged, but if you are someone's training partner you should consider how your language and actions are affecting not just you, but your tribe too. Just like finding your fitness fit and the right trainer, finding the right tribe and accountability partners is equally important. You don't necessarily have to hire a trainer or join a gym to find your tribe. Someone in your community may share your athletic goals, and if you find them your tribe can be born. Two people is a small tribe, and your tribe opens doors to two different networks of friends and family who may want to join you in your fitness pursuits.

A successful tribe or training partner will be like-minded, so you want to find people whose interests, goals, abilities, and dreams are similar to yours. Just as you did when considering a trainer, take some time to think about the important traits you want your tribe or training partner to possess. What matters to you?

Here are some traits that are important to me in finding a tribe member or training partner:

- They have a positive attitude.
- They are goal-oriented.
- They are committed.
- Their schedule is compatible with mine.
- Their fitness level is similar to mine.
- They are good company.

It is a good idea to interview your potential tribe or training partner, though in a less formal way than with your trainer. I have thrown in the towel several times because I was working with the wrong people or the wrong training partners, and that only prolonged my journey to living my athletic dreams.

I'VE BELONGED TO many tribes. Fifteen years ago at my first run club I found people who had the same goals as I did. On off days, when we weren't at the clinic, we would meet up and do our homework runs together. We were all new to running and excited about conquering the 5K distance and upcoming race. We had a common goal and were all enthusiastic about it. The members of this group were people I could talk to about my fitness dreams. Remember, up until that point I didn't have any tribe members interested in fitness, only a wine-drinking tribe I'd grown out of.

More recently, at my open-water swim clinic, my tribe consisted of nine other swimmers new to the open water, and while we would wait to start our session we would bob up and down in the lake and talk about races we wanted to do. We would share information about triathlons—which ones were good for beginner open-water swimmers—and talk about our fears and what worked to overcome them. These people understood why someone would train for months on end simply to cross a finish line. I felt part of the triathlon community and that sense of belonging only fueled my persistence to go further in the sport.

## The Team

ON YOUR ATHLETIC journey, your body may require maintenance. Over time, as your athletic goals expand, you may need
certain professionals to provide you with additional support
along the way. Over the years my own Rolodex has included
a list of supportive health professionals: a chiropractor, a massage therapist, a podiatrist, and a physician. I refer to them as
my team.

At times I've sought chiropractic help to align my body
because my hip or back was feeling out of alignment. I've
hired a massage therapist, my favorite of all team members,
to ease particularly sore muscles and help me get back on the
road to running. I've gone to a podiatrist to examine my gait,
and he provided some insoles that helped my feet strike properly for running and thus diminished the pain in my hip. Seeing
a skilled professional can clear up nagging pains quickly. Not
everyone will need additional team support, but for many people living a fully active life means at some point needing to
access professional help.

You won't likely need all your team members at once,
but it's important to be able to source the right people when
necessary.

I've built solid relationships with my team members, and
they've taken the time to understand my goals, support me in
achieving them, and share in my philosophy that health can be
achieved in a range of body sizes. Depending on your needs
your team might also include a nutritionist, an acupuncturist,
a naturopath, or other specialists.

These relationships can be close ones, as some of the work
these professionals do requires hands-on contact, or knowledge of your personal information. You may feel vulnerable, so
you must be sure to choose a team that you feel comfortable

with who can provide the support you need. Apply your CEO interviewing skills for your team members as well. You are in charge and only work with the best of the best, and that includes people you feel comfortable with.

## FINDING YOUR TEAM

Get recommendations from people you trust. If you ask your trainers and tribes, you will likely find a professional that suits the bill. Because you have already created a network of trainers that work from a weight neutral position and your tribe shares your goals and philosophy, they will likely be able to make the right suggestions. The Internet is also a good place to find professionals; however, it is important that you read the reviews for each practitioner.

I have found my team members by both referral and Internet research. The referrals have come from people I trust who understand my philosophy toward health and fitness. This is always the best way to find the right people. But when I am left to find a service provider by going in cold and doing online research I make sure to read their "About" page or staff bios. This gives me a sense of their philosophy, lifestyle, and accreditations.

Consider what is important to you. What will make you feel safe and comfortable? When you need a team member for body maintenance you will have already thought this through and you'll be ready to make the right choices. I want to save you from any kind of Dr. Brown Town experience.

---

**Zig Ziglar, motivational speaker:**
"The core of success is love, and that includes loving yourself enough to take care of yourself."

---

I HAVE BUILT a relationship based on trust with my team of professionals. Here are some of the traits I look for:

- They listen intently to my concerns.
- They create solid action plans.
- They are professional and punctual.
- They are personable and friendly.
- They treat you with an unbiased and judgment-free approach.
- They create an environment of comfort and ease.
- Their professional space is clean.
- They make getting appointments fairly easy with reasonable notice.

Remember that you deserve the best service providers and professionals on your team. Your dreams and your health are worth the effort required to put together your trainers, tribe, and team. You are in a position of power, and you don't have to engage with people who don't support your journey. And if a relationship with someone does not work out, do not hesitate to fire them. You are the head honcho.

**Lena Dunham, actress:**
"My mother raised me to believe that choice—the freedom to decide what you want to do with your life, how you want to be perceived and treated, to dress and act and engage the world in whatever way feels most natural, safe, and kind to you—was not a privilege but a right."

# FOUR

# Gear and Go Time

INDING THE RIGHT fitness gear can be an intimidating and overwhelming process.

The Internet is filled with pages of clothing, accessories, and equipment you may or may not need to start a new activity. You want to show up looking and feeling prepared—nobody wants to feel out of place—but how do you know what is essential for comfort and safety, and what is unnecessary? Where do you even start? Many people who are confused about what gear to buy may use it as a reason to give up the whole idea of exercise. I fully acknowledge that sourcing plus-size athletic apparel can be difficult—but don't give up!

I get it. My very first day at a mid-winter running clinic I showed up in wide-legged cropped yoga pants. I flapped along in the wind (and froze) next to more savvy runners in tight-fitting leggings. I had no idea. I knew I was going to be active, so I picked something from my closet that looked like "active-wear." My pants rode up between my legs as I ran, meaning I constantly had to stop and pull them down from my crotch. That night when we returned to the running store, I took a pair of tights from the rack and bought them immediately. They were worth every penny.

The initial investment in gear for a new activity can seem prohibitive, but in the long run, outfitting yourself properly pays off. Think of it not as an investment in a pair of running shoes but as an investment in your health and happiness. I think that is money well spent.

Through trial and error I have developed a list of gear must-haves. These are items that, with a few exceptions, should be relevant no matter what the activity.

## Seven Fitness Must-Haves

### 1. A GOOD SPORTS BRA

Two female runners designed the very first sports bra in 1977; they made it by sewing two jock straps together. Fortunately, the design and functionality have evolved quite a bit since then. All female athletes should invest in a good sports bra that fits comfortably and gives you good breast support.

The CBC has reported that more than 80 percent of women wear the wrong-sized bra.[1] An ill-fitting bra can be uncomfortable or even painful, and can wreak havoc when you exercise. Breasts are mostly composed of fatty tissue and are supported mainly by skin and fragile ligaments. These ligaments are not elastic, so during rigorous or high-impact sports, the breasts' bouncing pulls the ligaments, forcing them to stretch. A good sports bra can restrict this bounce by up to 60 percent. Although not true for every Big Fit Girl, many of us have very large breasts, so it is even more important to have the right support.

There are some important things to consider when purchasing a sports bra, especially if your "girls" are large. Find a bra that has wide, cushioned shoulder straps with a structured fabric rather than a stretchy fabric design that has a lot of give. You want some stretch at the rib band to secure the bra, but not in the cup.

I have owned many sports bras and have found that unless a sports apparel company has designed them, they don't provide enough support. Some brands known for offering the most support to plus-size women include Enell Sports Bra, Under Armour, Panache Sports Bra, and Lane Bryant's Livi Active line.

## 2. ATHLETIC SHOES

When buying shoes to support your athletic efforts, look at functionality over fashion. You need to find the right shoe for the right sport, and it must fit properly.

Because we all come with different-shaped feet, different body alignment, and different gaits, different brands and styles will fit your feet better than others. I may lean toward a certain shoe because it looks good, but need a wider shoe to support my feet for running. I have had good luck with New Balance and Mizuno, but a different brand might be right for you.

There are three categories of running shoes, one for each type of gait. Your gait is largely determined by the anatomy of your foot and the biomechanics of your unique body. If your gait includes pronation, the arch of your foot flattens during your stride, causing your foot and ankle to roll inward. In contrast, supination occurs when you have high arches, causing your foot to roll outward. When your foot strikes the ground, it doesn't have much cushion. Because the foot doesn't flatten on impact, there is little shock absorption, causing you to favor the outside of your foot. People with feet that have an average arch usually have the most efficient and effective gait without added support, referred to as a neutral foot. In this gait, the foot strikes without pronation or supination.

The good news is there are specific types of shoes designed to meet the needs of these three gaits. The right type of shoe provides the foundation for an injury-free athletic experience.

To find out where you fit in these three categories, you need to have a proper shoe fitting. Athletic shoe retailers—in particular, specialty running stores—often offer a free foot analysis to make sure you find the right fit. During the analysis, trained store staff will watch you walk a straight line. In some stores they may ask you to walk on a treadmill at different inclines. Sometimes the staff will ask you to squat to see how your feet stay positioned while you are performing exercises. When you squat, your feet may roll out or in slightly, and this tells a story about your specific body mechanics and how your foot responds to certain movements. Some stores have a heat-sensored foot-impression plate that shows the exact points your feet strike when you walk or stand.

I recommend that all my clients get fitted properly for a good quality pair of shoes. When your feet are happy, you are happy! Shoes that fit or support your foot poorly may cause numbness, toenail damage, blisters, and more chronic injuries to your heels or foot fascia. Your health and fitness, and your ability to reach your goals, are worth the trip to the running store to get fitted properly to avoid injury. Remember, shoes also wear out with mileage. Regular runners should replace their shoes every 300 to 500 miles (or 500 to 800 km). For example, if you're doing three 5K runs per week a loose guide would be to replace your shoes after a year, while for three 10K runs per week, you'll need to replace your shoes every four to six months.

JEN MCLELLAN IS a plus-size runner and the founder of Plus Size Birth. On her popular blog, along with her writings on plus-size pregnancy, Jen also writes about her fitness pursuits to inspire her audience to adopt an active lifestyle both pre- and post-pregnancy. In a recent interview she talked to me about her first experience getting properly fitted for shoes:

When I started my journey to begin running, my greatest fear was hurting myself. That is, until I learned that being properly fitted for running shoes meant I needed to run on a treadmill in a shoe store. It was pretty much my worst nightmare. I imagined people stopping what they were doing to stare and laugh at me. As you can imagine, I was a big ball of nerves when I finally built up the confidence to get properly fitted. It turns out all of my fears were completely off base. No one laughed, and the salesperson was super encouraging of my desire to run. The results of my ten-second jog on the treadmill were pretty cool. I found out I have great balance! On that day I not only found the perfect running shoes but also overcame a big fear of running in public. That experience gave me a lot of confidence and catapulted me forward in my running journey.

I know it seems intimidating; walking into a specialty store devoted to runners may make you feel overwhelmed and self-conscious. But like Jen did, you will find that most salespeople are happy to help you. You may even discover a player for your master team!

### 3. HYDRATION TOOLS

It may seem obvious, but consuming enough fluids during a workout is very important. Not doing so can cause dehydration. The symptoms of dehydration can include dizziness, headache, and fatigue. When you lose or use more fluid than you take in, your body won't have enough water to carry out its normal functions.

Proper hydration begins before you even start exercising. You need to keep yourself hydrated throughout each day, and even more so on days when you plan to exercise. If you are a morning exerciser, it is a good idea to take in some water before and during your workout. But if you have been practicing good hydration day to day, you will be hydrated enough for your morning workouts already. If it is hot out or you are working out in a hot environment or for long periods of time, you will lose fluids at a faster rate through sweating and you will be more prone to dehydration.

There are a few types of gear that can help you stay hydrated while you are exercising.

The most common is, of course, a really good large water bottle. The bottle is most convenient when you can set it aside in the gym or on the court or put it in your bike bottle holder. There are all kinds of water bottles on the market today, from plastic insulated bottles and bottles with built-in straws to environmentally friendly glass water bottles and stainless steel bottles. Selling water bottles as a fitness accessory has become a lucrative business, with bottles ranging from $2.00 all the way up to $50.00.

Hydration belts are commonly found in running stores and consist of a thin belt with small bottles attached (usually three or four evenly distributed on the belt). These belts generally come in conventional sizing, but extenders can be purchased to fit a range of waist sizes. These are especially useful when you are walking, running, or hiking.

A hydration pack, which can be worn on your back like a backpack, contains a bladder, a clear bag that you can fill with water that closes with a heavy-duty ziplock closure. It comes in various sizes that hold up to three liters of water. A tube that extends from the bladder and clips onto the shoulder strap allows for easy reach and drinking.

Hikers, cyclists, skiers, snowboarders, and endurance runners often use a hydration pack because it allows them to carry large amounts of water that they can drink on the go with little effort.

## 4. ATHLETIC JACKET

If you live in a climate that includes snow or rain, an athletic jacket will become one of the most valuable items in your wardrobe. A good athletic jacket should be easy to move in, water-resistant, and breathable. The best jackets for outdoor fitness are built for sweating and control your temperature. They are usually made from a polyester blend, since polyester is inherently quick-drying and water-repellent; it absorbs only one-tenth as much water as nylon and reduces interior condensation. If you are willing to spend more money on a jacket, you can look at Gore-Tex options, which are waterproof, wind resistant, and breathable (but not necessary).

Since I live in a rainforest, I am pretty attached to my running jacket. Inclement weather can't keep me at home.

Find a jacket that has the look, feel, and fit that best suits you. Mine has zippers at the armpits, a nice but not necessary technical feature that offers breathability and allows me to manage my body temperature without taking the jacket off in the rain. It also helps me manage body temperature by releasing heat and moisture.

As with all athletic clothing for big girls, plus-size running jackets can be hard to find. If my clients are having a difficult time finding a good running jacket in their size, I have recommended that they look at men's running jackets as a last resort. Whenever possible, however, I urge you to put in some time to find a jacket specifically for women. Although men's and women's running jackets may look fairly similar, they usually fit quite differently. Men's jackets tend to be longer in the arms and torso, so while a men's jacket may fit around your midsection the rest of it may look oversized.

To help you avoid looking like you raided your dad's closet, at the end of the chapter I've listed twenty-two places where you can find plus-size athletic apparel.

## 5. COMPRESSION PANTS OR RUNNING TIGHTS

Compression pants may be a necessity for some athletes. Some of us have more body fat on our lower half or stomach—this may bounce during exercise, which can be uncomfortable. Compression pants take care of the bounce that can occur in high-impact sports (like running) by holding your body in place and compressing the skin to reduce the movement while you are exercising.

Wearing compression garments has become popular, and many major brands have jumped on board this trend. They also make big promises in their marketing messages. Adidas says its TechFit line "focuses your muscle energy to generate maximum explosive power, acceleration and long-term endurance." Under Armour says its leggings "deliver increased power and stamina."

Despite all the promises, my recommendation comes from an understanding that compression pants may provide comfort rather than big gains in performance. If you feel any discomfort around your bum or legs while exercising, try a pant with compression. But a good running tight or athletic legging may be all you need. Much of finding the right gear is about trial and error and what works for you and your body.

## 6. MOISTURE-WICKING WORKOUT TOPS

I often see plus-size women working out in big cotton t-shirts. I don't blame them. There isn't much selection of cutting edge fitness apparel in larger sizes that is readily available in-store. I have had my challenges, and I know not finding your size can be discouraging. Although cotton is not my first choice, you can get away with wearing it for your indoor workout. But if you are an outdoor fitness enthusiast, you should invest in fabrics that wick moisture away from the skin.

These fabrics will help you manage your body temperature.

When a fabric is absorbent, like cotton, the moisture fills the fabric and sits on your skin. If you are outdoors, this moisture against your skin will make you feel cold. In contrast, a fabric that pulls moisture away from the body will make you feel more comfortable.

The material used in athletic apparel has become extremely advanced (and expensive). There are a few fabric blends you can buy at a lower price point, however. Synthetic materials like polyester, polyethylene, and microfiber-based fabrics are less expensive than most other blends and have excellent water-wicking properties. Wool, in particular merino wool, is more costly but has excellent water and odor repelling properties and is especially good for cold or wet climates.

In lower temperatures, consider a moisture-wicking base layer and an athletic jacket to keep you warm and dry.

### 7. CHAFING CREAM

You may have heard of the term "chub rub." It refers to that serious discomfort you experience when the skin between your legs, between the butt cheeks, or under your arms or breasts rubs together. This rub, or chafing, causes a burn-like rash as the skin repeatedly comes into contact with other skin. It is very uncomfortable and in more extreme cases can cause blistering and scarring. So unless you have a thigh gap, listen up!

You may find chafing becomes a particular problem in hot climates or during the summer as moist skin rubs together. I've also experienced chafing from running in the rain.

You can reduce the chance of chafing by taking such measures as removing tags from bras and ensuring that the seam stitching in pants is not too prominent: the less prominent the seam, the less chance of chafing. And a liberal application of chafing cream goes a long way toward protecting the skin. I generously apply chafing cream when cycling long distances and when running. If you are heading out for a short distance or going to the gym, you may not need chafing cream. But it might be a good idea to keep it on hand, especially in humid summer weather. Some brands to consider are Glide, 2Toms, and Chamois Butt'r cream. Some people use less conventional chafing creams and go for products they already have, like anti-perspirant or Vaseline.

2Toms published an official list of chafing zones of the body: between the arms and sides of the body, between the upper thighs, the groin area, the nipples, the back of the heels, the tops of the toes. If you are a triathlete and wearing a wetsuit, I've also heard of people applying creams around their neck under the collar of the wetsuit.

Fitness apparel and equipment are industries worth billions of dollars, and there are innumerable products to choose from. You can find anything from technical gadgets that allow you to listen to music underwater while you swim to sports watches that track calories, heart rate, elevation gains, and sleep patterns, and will even yell at you if you are sedentary for too long. You can certainly go crazy with gear to support your athletic life, but these essentials are the best places to start.

Beyond the basic needs there is a whole slew of items specific to certain sports. While you won't need all of these items, here is a list you might consider if you plan to extensively participate in any of the following activities:

**Running**
Running socks
Shoes
Running jacket
Running tights
Running bra
Moisture wicking shirt
Hydration belt

**Yoga**
Yoga mat
Straps
Blocks
Water bottle
Towel

**Cycling**
Helmet
Padded cycling shorts
Cycling gloves
Water bottle
Cycling jersey
Anti-glare sunglasses

**Weight Training**
Cross-training shoes
Training gloves
Water bottle

**Boxing**
Boxing gloves
Hand wraps
Pro-pads or target

**Walking or Hiking**
Walking or hiking shoes
Walking or hiking poles
Backpack
Hydration pack or bottle

**Swimming**
Goggles
Swim cap
Sport swimsuit
Training flippers

## Things to Consider When Gearing Up

### GEAR IS AN INVESTMENT

Good gear doesn't always come cheap. You might need to commit to an initial investment to start a new activity. There are some things you can buy cheaply, but I recommend splurging on certain items for your safety and comfort.

Spend the money on running or athletic shoes. Your feet need the best support possible and require a good fit. The same is true for sports bras. I've tried to go cheap on a sports bra, and the result was not enough support. A good bra is essential for the comfort of your back and breasts and for the enjoyment of your sessions. Bouncing all over the place is never fun, so make the investment.

A good running jacket can be hard to come by at a lower cost. When apparel is cheaply made the garment is usually less breathable and your sweat and body heat will stay under the jacket. Remember wearing a K-Way jacket as a kid? Less breathability often comes with odor. We don't want that—hot and stinky isn't our goal. Make an investment in a jacket. I promise you will be happy you did.

Cheaper is fine for running tights or compression pants, but when you spent more, the quality generally increases. Some chain stores, like Old Navy, offer good pants at low prices. Higher-end athletic apparel companies offer a better pant that is more breathable with less odor, but to get started you don't need to spend a bunch of money on the best.

Cheaper is fine for athletic shirts too. Moisture-wicking shirts will always be priced higher than cotton shirts, but they don't have to be expensive. You can find retailers that offer reasonably priced athletic shirts, and cotton is also fine as you get started. I want you geared up and ready to go but I don't want budget to get in the way, so stick to less expensive shirts in the beginning.

If you are a swimmer, you don't need a high-performance swimsuit or triathlon suit at first. They can be really expensive, and while you are getting started an investment here likely won't change your performance. Find something you feel comfortable in and save your money for down the road. Keep some of your budget for a good pair of goggles that won't leak or fog easily.

### FINDING PLUS-SIZE GEAR CAN BE CHALLENGING

The fitness apparel market doesn't recognize the plus-size community as target consumers, so it is often difficult to find clothes that fit larger athletes, especially in-store. But as the media begin to show plus-size people engaged in sports and as more of us demand workout apparel tailored to our needs, this is starting to change. New plus-size clothing companies are popping up monthly. However, many clothing options that include plus sizes are only available online. Until we can get retailers to step up and make apparel readily available in-store, here are a few tips to remember when buying online.

Most online shopping sites will include information about how their clothing fits. Look for a sizing chart that matches body measurements with a size. This isn't a guarantee of a good fit, but it is a guideline. Most size charts use three measurements: bust, hips, and waist. Remember, your bust should be measured at your nipple line, your hips are the widest part of your body, and your waist is the narrowest point. Keep your measurements handy when you shop.

Find out what real customers think of the products before you buy. In online reviews, customers will often comment on whether the clothing fits big, small, or true to size, and of course if they are displeased with a particular quality of the clothing. Their comments might raise a red flag.

Check out a retailer on their social channels to see what images they are sharing or others are sharing for them. For example, on Instagram, use the hashtag #torridfashion to see pictures of everyday people wearing the brand Torrid's clothing.

When I find an item I really love, I like to stock up! You never know when the item will be out-of-stock or when styles will change.

## FINDING YOUR FIT

Not all plus-size bodies are the same—we all have different shapes. Sometimes finding the best clothing for you will require trial and error. This is where reviews and photos, on a plus-size clothing company's website and on social media, can really help. Before buying online, be sure you understand the company's return policy.

Some retailers do not cater to all sizes. Remember Lululemon founder Chip Wilson's infamous statement about his company's yoga pants? "They don't work for some women's bodies." And maybe you caught what Mike Jeffries, formerly of Abercrombie & Fitch, said in *Salon:* "A lot of people don't belong [in our clothes], and they can't belong. Are we exclusionary? Absolutely."

These statements might make you angry; I've felt that way too. But you can't change everyone's mind. Instead, spend your money at retailers that create a great product for a range of sizes. You can find fantastic retailers out there that provide quality and fashionable apparel for plus-size women. Here are my trusted favorites:

**TWENTY-TWO RESOURCES FOR PLUS-SIZE ACTIVE APPAREL**

1. *Livi Active Line by Lane Bryant* Offers a range of styles of tanks, graphic tees, and hoodies, sizes 14–26. Available in store or at *lanebryant.com.*
2. *Athleta by Gap* Great basic workout wear in a huge variety of styles and colors. Sizes XXS–2X. Available at *athleta.gap.com.*
3. *Lola Getts* Offers fashion-forward performance apparel in sizes 14–24. Workout basics that keep it classy with a simple, three-color palette (black, white, and gray). *lolagetts.com*
4. *JunoActive* Offers a wide selection of activewear in sizes XL–6X. JunoActive believes that every woman deserves to be active and that to be active you need the clothes to do it in! *junonia.com*
5. *Katie K Active* Workout gear that looks and feels amazing on women sizes small–3X. As a fitness trainer, Katie Kozloff worked with women and heard first hand their opinions on what was lacking in the activewear industry. *katiekactive.com*
6. *Superfit Hero* A size-inclusive brand of high-performance activewear for women sizes XS–3XL. *superfithero.com*
7. *Female for Life* Specializes in maternity sportswear and lifestyle sportswear in sizes 6–24. *femaleforlife.com.au*

8. *Fullbeauty Sport* The premier fashion destination for sizes 12+ with a mission to make you look and feel beautiful. *fullbeauty.com*

9. *Enell* Dedicated to providing women C cup and above with the opportunity to fully participate in an active lifestyle by offering state-of-the-art, high-quality performance sports bras 32C to 52G. *enell.com*

10. NOLA *Activewear by Addition Elle* Delivers modern, fashionable clothes. An inspiring, world-class shopping experience in-store & online. *additionelle.com*

11. *Old Navy* Offers fashionable, plus-size active apparel at an affordable price. *oldnavy.com*

12. *Manifesta* Offers curvy and athletic workout clothes for women sizes 0–28. *mymanifesta.com*

13. *Zella Plus-Size Workout Clothing for Women by Nordstrom* Combines innovative performance with a feminine edge. Zella gear fits perfectly into an active lifestyle without compromising on style. *shop.nordstrom.com*

14. *Active Zone by Penningtons* Penningtons advocates for body diversity and size acceptance in fashion and inspires and empowers women to find their own sense of style. Active Zone offers fashionable activewear. *www.penningtons.com*

15. REI An active lifestyle mecca, offering all you need for an active lifestyle. Products come in sizes 0–3X. *rei.com*

16. *Happy Puppies Athleticwear* Offers comfortable clothes designed to fit a wide range of women, sizes 0–30. *happy-puppies.myshopify.com*

17. *K-Deer Luxury Activewear* Luxury athletic clothing for the modern woman. High-quality fabric meets exceptional fit and durability. Made in the USA, sizes SM–4XL. *k-deer.com*

18. *Swimsuits for All* Offers a large selection of swimwear in plus sizes up to 34. Swimsuits for All offers bikinis, one pieces, and athletic suits for all your needs. *swimsuitsforall.com*

19. *Rainbeau Curves* Fashionable activewear that flatters a fuller figure using premium performance fabrics. *rainbeau.com*
20. *Nettle's Tale Swimwear* With a mission to provide what you want for your body, age, and style, offers swimwear in a variety of styles and sizes from xs–4x. *nettlestale.com*
21. *Torrid* Offers a range of fashionable, functional activewear in edgy, trendy styles for the active woman in sizes up to 6x. *torrid.com/active*
22. *Marika* Has been making colorful, fun activewear for women of all shapes and sizes since 1982. Their sizes range from xs–3x. *marika.com*

The right gear for you is out there. You just have to know where to look and how to go about finding the right fit. Happy sweating in your new gear!

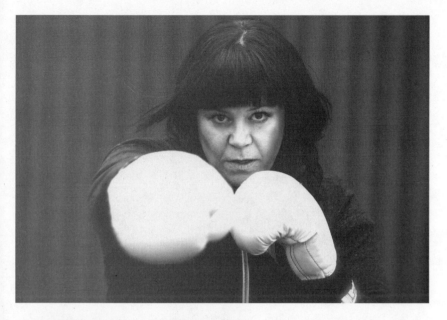

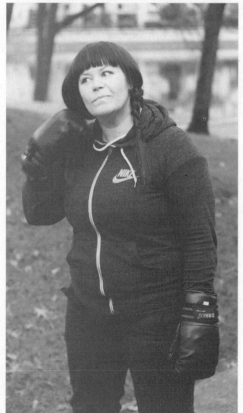

Boxing sessions on Granville
Island in Vancouver, BC.

PAUL DEANE

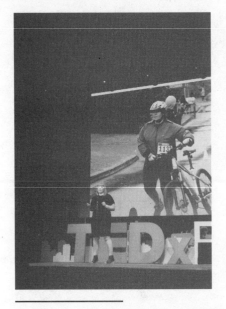
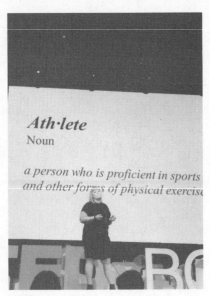

On the TEDx stage delivering the talk "Let's Think Again about Athleticism." TARRYN RUDOLPH

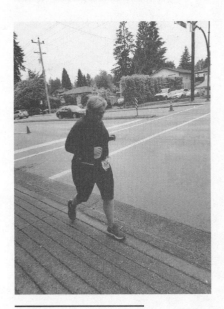
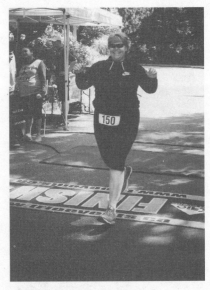

On-course at the North Shore Triathlon. PAULA ANDERSON

Crossing the finish line at the Creek Classic Triathlon.
PAULINE DEANE

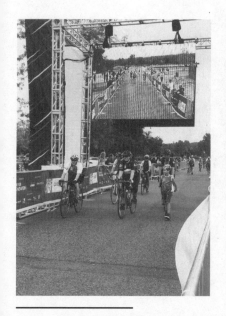
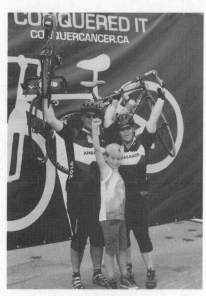

Fourth finish at the Ride to Conquer Cancer, a 250K cycle from Vancouver, BC, to Seattle, Washington, for the BC Cancer Foundation. PAULINE DEANE

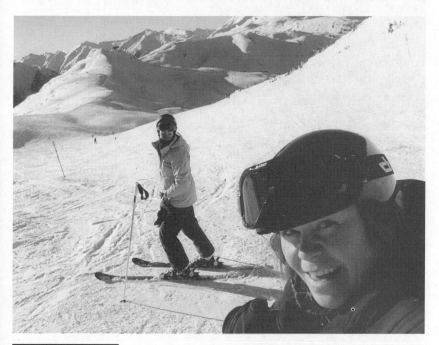

On Burnt Stew Trail, Whistler Mountain, BC, for an annual birthday ski with Hollie McBeth.

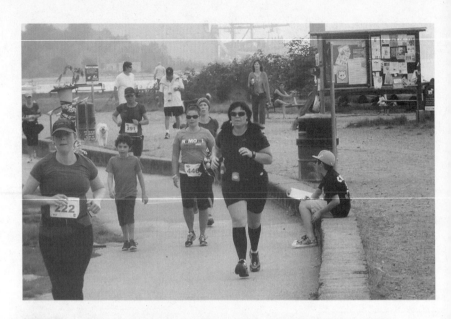

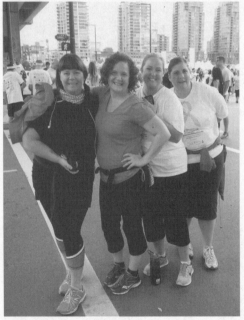

*above* On the 15K Coho Run approaching the finish line at Ambleside Beach, West Vancouver, BC.
JEANNIE BLAIN

*left* On the 5K Run for the Cure with Body Exchange clients, Vancouver, BC.

# FIVE

# Goals That Stick

AT KILOMETER 19 of 21 I was struggling to make it to the finish line. The runners around me looked like I felt— sluggish, exhausted, and ready to be done. When I thought I had nothing left to pull me through, I heard the sounds of the finish line: the band playing and the announcer's voice naming the finishers. A small voice in my head said, "You can *do* this." I dug deep and pulled out every ounce of energy I had left. I could visualize my finish and felt the power of sixteen weeks of training.

I pumped my arms, and my legs moved farther and faster. As I turned the corner, the finish line was in sight. My mind went into positive overdrive: "You can do it, you're almost there, *go, go, go!*" I looked down at my watch; I was running faster than I had all morning. This was my moment. The final kilometer.

I could see the people standing behind the barriers cheering me on, but I could no longer hear them. Everything had gone silent as I concentrated. I felt like a champion on the verge of victory as I laid everything I had out on the road and sprinted.

As my foot landed over the finish line, the noise rushed in, and I heard the crowd, the band, and my heavy breathing as I bent over, hands to knees, catching my breath. I heard the announcer call my name as I was ushered away from the finish line.

This day marked the completion of sixteen weeks of training and my third half-marathon.

As I rested and refueled, I reminded myself that getting here was not an accident. I worked hard and set clear goals.

To date I have completed four half-marathons, five triathlons, and four long-distance biking events, in addition to smaller accomplishments, and I have big plans for more.

I dream of summiting Mount Kilimanjaro, completing a Half Ironman (training in progress!), kayaking the Colorado River, running a full marathon, and hiking the West Coast Trail.

But none of it will happen unless I make a plan and put it into action. Goal setting has been the vehicle to all of my physical, entrepreneurial, and life achievements.

My goals have involved finish lines, but yours don't have to. Not everyone wants to run a half-marathon or bike in a long-distance race. Goals can be as simple as walking for ten minutes a day or as challenging as completing a triathlon. But it is important to have some goals, which act as building blocks to reaching your highest potential and limitless life.

---

**Unknown:**
"Life is short, fragile and does not wait for anyone. There will never be a perfect time to pursue your dreams and goals."

---

Don't rush things; start off with small steps. Every single athlete started with that first walk, run, or trip to the gym.

WENDY WELSHER IS a plus-size athlete and personal trainer from Sacramento, California. She started off with small goals, and over time her accomplishments grew.

One day, I had had enough of my unhealthy lifestyle. Of course the intimidation of the gym still haunted me, so I started working out at home. It was the first of many small goals that propelled me to where I am today. I began with simple aerobic games, running in place, and yoga on my Nintendo Wii. Instantly, I saw a change in myself, not just in my physical appearance but also in my overall well-being. My motivation started to take over those old habits, and I began to create small goals around eating for athletic performance, staying active, and staying away from the things and people that would trigger my unhealthy lifestyle. My confidence began to build with every healthier choice I made amongst so many negative choices in my path.

As this new woman emerged from within, I created more goals and challenges in my life. Accomplishing one goal acted as a building block for another. I found a trainer who made a huge impact on my life. Together we continued to set more attainable goals; she pushed me physically and mentally to be my very best. For the first time in my life, I was doing it. I had purpose and a sense of achievement.

LIKE ME, WENDY arrived at a place in her life where she had simply had enough. Until I was ready to change, my unhealthy behaviors served a purpose in my life. They allowed me to stay where I felt safe. Although my behaviors were hurting me, they were familiar and in that sense, comforting. I had never practiced goal setting and didn't realize then that not knowing where to start and how to find a path kept me in the same spot.

Since my own transformation, I have learned there are common stages to human change. We can only really set sound goals when we are ready to do so. Our goals can't be what others want for us; we must be psychologically ready to set them.

These are the five stages of change. Take a moment to consider where you might be in these five stages. It will help you determine your readiness to commit to your goals.

## The Five Stages of Change

### STAGE ONE: PRE-CONTEMPLATION

In this stage you aren't yet ready to change your habits. You don't yet recognize the patterns you need to break. This stage is also referred to as "denial." I was in this stage for many years. I thought I was a "free spirit," and I used this excuse to maintain a reckless life marked by self-destructive habits.

It's difficult for others to reach you in the pre-contemplation stage: you aren't open to the idea of change, and your unwillingness keeps you closed off to new ways of life. At this stage, you may not even know what is possible. You are operating in a state of unawareness.

This was the case for Australian plus-size runner Carin McCoy.

Until Carin unexpectedly signed up for a 5K run, she had no desire to get active or change anything in her life. Carin wasn't aware that her life could be improved by getting active. The result of her doing the race ignited a new outlook on life and shifted her into action for the long-term.

I became ready to move into action when my two young sons were struggling with their health. At the time my toddler and six-month-old were diagnosed with a genetic condition. We had been spending a lot of time at the children's hospital, and obviously, I was really stressed. I felt like I had no control of the situation. The hospital organized an annual fun run, "Run for the Kids," and even though I was the most unathletic person I knew, I also knew I had to be part of it for my kids. I trained my rather large butt off and was so proud that I, ever so slowly, completed the 5K fun run without stopping. I experienced a runners' high and realized my body did have the fight in it to lead an athletic lifestyle even though I didn't fit the stereotypical picture of an athlete. I am plus-size and I too have the genetic condition passed on to my sons. While I was out running, all the stress of those hospital visits melted away; [I realized] it was exactly the therapy I needed.

Carin realized her athletic potential by putting the needs of her sons first. The twist in her journey was that in putting someone else first, she was finally taking care of herself.

Often there is an event or end-point that pulls people out of this stage. When I decided to make changes I was at an emotional rock bottom; that was my end-point. I hated everything about my life and I *had* to change. Some people make changes because of a death in the family or kids moving out of the house and discovering there is now time for more activity. Or a health-related diagnosis can motivate someone to seek more exercise. The hunger for change is an opportunity to sit up and listen, and see what might be possible. Because you have this book in your hands, you are clearly ready (if you haven't advanced even further) to hit this next stage.

### STAGE TWO: CONTEMPLATION

In contemplation you are willing to consider that changing your behavior might be beneficial, but you are still thinking it through and haven't yet committed to action.

I know this stage well. I wanted to change for years but didn't do anything about it until things got unbearable and I was unhappy enough to be ready. You might be able to relate to this. It's like a tango dance with the transition of change: one step forward, one step back until one day you're ready to go all in.

Many people who inquire about my program are at this stage. They are curious but remain unsure and are weighing the cost and the time and energy commitment of going all in. Remember reckless fitness girl invading my body? That was me getting dragged across the line into the next stage of change. I think of reckless fitness girl every day because someone may remain in contemplation for months, or even years, or may never find the motivation to advance.

You must have a motivating belief behind your desire for change. If a person has a death in the family, their motivating belief might be that exercise will improve their health and contribute to their own longevity. In my case, I was incredibly unhappy and knew that an athletic lifestyle was the polar opposite of the one I was living. My motivating belief was that getting active would take me far away from that life and I would finally find happiness. I believed that to my core, and it motivated my change.

We often have family members that suggest we need to change, but if we decide to change for the sake of others, we lack a deep-rooted belief to motivate us. Although family members often mean well, it has to come from within if we want the change to last.

For example, if you tell your doctor you've been feeling crappy lately, he or she may tell you to get some exercise. It won't actually happen until you have assumed the belief that exercise is the answer to feeling good. Only then will you have the desire to make the necessary changes. Someone in pre-contemplation would likely not heed this advice, but a contemplator has opened the door to others' suggestions and may consider them.

One of my core values is that exercise is a vital part of daily living. It is my lifeline to physical and mental health, and without it I have the potential to slip into a dark place. I believe this to the core, and it motivates me every single day. My core belief about exercise keeps me motivated for the long-term, but as you know it hasn't always been that way for me. When I was in my twenties, I did not have a core motivating belief about exercise, so I never exercised for more than a couple of weeks. I wanted to lose weight; at the time my core motivating belief was that thinness would bring me happiness, and when thinness involved being hungry all the time, I couldn't stick to my goal.

Do you have a motivating belief behind your desire to change? If you do, that is very encouraging because it will help move you to the next stage.

### STAGE THREE: PREPARATION

In this stage you are aware that you need to change; you are ready to do it, but you need to first prepare yourself mentally, and often physically, for the action required. In preparation you may start by calling friends to see if they want to meet you at the gym or join you in starting a new fitness program. You begin recruiting your master team, maybe interviewing trainers. And you start thinking about what your plan of attack will be.

This is an exciting stage, and one I enjoy being in myself. When I entered my first triathlon, preparing for the training was new and exciting. I was never a strong swimmer, so this stage included watching YouTube videos of various swimming techniques that I would then incorporate in the pool. I learned how to transition from the pool to the bike and the bike to the run by watching videos of pro triathletes. I reached out to friends who had completed triathlons and asked for training plans that I could review against my own schedule. The preparation phase gave me energy and enthusiasm.

### STAGE FOUR: ACTION

Action is where the magic happens. You have worked up the courage to walk out the door on the first day of a new running program or dance class or aerobics class. If you are running, you lace up your shoes for the very first time and hit the road to start the training program you have been planning. During this stage it is normal to encounter fear. When the fear feels overwhelming, stay focused on why you are doing this—the core belief that got you started on this path in the first place. What is driving you toward a different life? Answer this question and you will always know your "why." Your "why" is your driving motivator, your core belief for change, and what ignites the desire to make changes in your life. Having a strong "why," and regularly reminding yourself of it can be the difference between faltering and letting go of your goals and sticking to your vision. Rehearse your "why" in your head often, and keep your eyes on the prize.

### STAGE FIVE: MAINTENANCE

Maintenance is continued action. You must continually set goals and update them, check your progress, and tweak your plan. I think about the things I want to accomplish months in advance. At the start of the year I already know what I am training for over the next twelve months and have planned out how to do it. However, life happens and sometimes plans need to be adjusted. To stay on track it's important to make a plan, and as each month begins, to review the plan and adjust dates and times if necessary. Making a plan and allowing for changes to it will help you avoid a last-minute bail. Maintaining a new behavior is the most challenging part of any change in lifestyle. It also requires continued accountability—you need to have a plan, show up, and remember why you started. Don't let yourself slide back into contemplation when you feel tired or discouraged or slip into pre-contemplation, thinking that you don't really need to make changes.

When things get tough you might conclude that you need to get back to "safe" ground. Are you afraid to fail? Are you afraid to go outside of your comfort zone? You need to remain positive and fixed on your new commitment. A great way to do this is to create a vision board that shows your desired outcomes. Remember when we talked about visualization and imagery earlier in the book? A vision board is another tool to keep your goal in your line of sight. It is also a way to remember why you started your fitness journey.

A vision board is a collage of images, pictures, and affirmations. Creating a vision board can be a useful tool to help you conceptualize your goals and can serve as a source of motivation as you work toward achieving them. The greatest thing is that *you* get to decide how you want your life to look; it's life by design. You can also post affirming messages to yourself around your home and workspace. Seeing these positive messages on a daily basis reaffirms those ideas in our minds.

I've talked about the lack of positive messaging and imagery for plus-size women in mainstream media, but we can supply that in our own spaces; it's up to us to create our own messaging. We need to constantly reinforce the idea that our dreams absolutely can become reality, and imagery and positive messages will do that.

In my own story, continued success hinged on short-term goals and small wins. My small wins consisted of just getting to the run club. I wasn't focused on pace, distance, or anything else; at first it was just about showing up. Then I focused on getting my homework runs done too. That was more manageable than, right off the bat, looking at the big picture of running a full 5K. I took each day one at a time, and I just focused on the training that was required that day. When you are rewarded with a feeling of success because you made it through that spin class or reached that next light post on your run, you are less likely to throw in the towel when things get harder. It's the small wins that will carry you to the big picture goal, every time.

Here are some strategies to get you through even the tough stuff.

## Goal Setting 101

WHEN I TRAINED to become a fitness professional, I learned the concepts around setting concrete and attainable goals. When asked, many of my clients express hopes instead of more tangible goals. Hopes may be what we ultimately want, but without clearly mapping out how to achieve our hopes, they will likely remain just that.

I often hear clients say things like this: "I want to lose fifty pounds because I have my cousin's wedding coming up this summer." If I follow up and ask, "What is your nutrition and fitness plan for making this happen?" I am usually met with silence. People have great intentions, but many lack the tools to clearly identify how to reach their goals. To assist them, they can use a system like the SMART goal setting principle, which breaks down the goal mapping process. SMART is an acronym for Specific, Measurable, Attainable, Realistic, and Timely. It is highly effective in creating solid, achievable goals in fitness and in life. Here are the principles behind SMART goal setting.

## THE SMART BREAKDOWN

### Specific

A non-specific goal sounds like this: "I plan to go to the gym this year." Are you ready to seize this goal by the horns? It doesn't sound like it. Nor does it sound like you have a proper plan in place for how to make this happen. For years, I had non-specific goals. They were more like dreams that never materialized. Back then I didn't know about SMART goal setting. A more specific goal would be: "I am going to go to the gym this year, three times a week for one hour each session."

### Measurable

Planning to go to the gym doesn't have any measurable outcomes attached to it.

Goals should be results-focused, and that's where the measurable component comes in. For example: "I am going to go to the gym this year, three times a week for one hour each session. My goal is to be able to run on the treadmill for thirty minutes straight." This goal now has measurable markers. The measure doesn't have to be competitive, like completing a race or event. It can be anything measurable that shows progression.

### Attainable

Goals must be attainable, and the SMART system reminds you to stay within the parameters of what is possible for you. I recommend small goals to start with. If you haven't exercised in years, the goal "I am going to exercise six days a week for an hour each time" might be difficult to maintain. Your ambition is admirable, but you may risk setting yourself up for failure or injury. We live in an "instant" culture, and people tend to set unattainable goals because they want the instant results they see promised everywhere. The truth is, attainable goal-setting means setting goals that you are likely to meet, within certain timelines, with the knowledge that there are no instant results.

When I started my fitness journey, my first goal was to just show up two times a week to my running group. For someone who may have been sedentary for many years, the goal of showing up to the gym two to three times a week is enough to start. A good way of making sure your goal is attainable is breaking down how you will achieve it. Such as: "I am going to go to the gym three days a week. For the first month I am going to run on the treadmill for fifteen minutes. The next month I will increase that time to twenty minutes and the next to the full thirty minutes." You now know this goal is attainable within three months.

Trying to do too much too quickly is a good way to become discouraged if you can't follow through or if you become overwhelmed by the enormity of the commitment involved. Doing too much too fast may lead to injury and derail your plan entirely.

Your attainable goal will be different from someone else's; you need to begin from where you are now. That also means not comparing yourself to others or what you used to be able to do before kids, in your twenties, or even last year. The only thing relevant to setting attainable goals today is where you are starting from now.

---

**Theodore Roosevelt, 26th president of the United States:**
"Comparison is the thief of joy."

---

### Realistic
Realistic goals are goals you are likely to meet. Sometimes people are confused about how a realistic goal differs from

an attainable goal. Here's an example: A client's goal this year may be to go to the gym for seven sessions a week for the next six months. While going to the gym seven days a week could be attainable—it *could* be done—is it realistic to think that this is something that could be sustained? It's not really realistic to try to manage a workout regime every day without any rest days. Same goes for someone who wants to run a 5K race. That goal is totally attainable, but it's not realistic to think that you can get off the couch and run a 5K by next weekend. The realistic component of the goal setting is to set goals that we have a good chance of meeting. Starting with unrealistic goals will feel discouraging and may cause you to throw in the towel.

Over time our bodies change, as do commitments to our family and career. If you work full-time, a rigorous training schedule might not work for you. You might, however, find it reasonable to take running shoes to work and walk or run for thirty minutes during your lunch hour. Your exercise regime has to work with your life or it will, for sure, go out the window.

Always consider your lifestyle, the time you have available to you, and your current physical abilities.

**Timely**
When you don't attach a time frame to a goal, it lives in the forever realm of "someday." We all have those "someday" dreams, but they often remain dreams simply because we haven't attached a concrete timeline or schedule to achieving them. We plan social events, dentist appointments, and shopping trips; shouldn't we make room in our calendars for pursuing our deepest desires?

As an example of setting a timeline to your goals, you might say: "I am going to go to the gym three days a week, for one hour a day. During that time I will work on building my time on the treadmill, starting with fifteen minutes, and will also do other strength-training activities. Within three months my goal is to run on the treadmill for thirty minutes without stopping."

Now the goal of "planning to go to the gym this year" has become SMART. It is measurable, attainable, realistic, and has a time frame attached to it. This is SMART goal setting.

I recommend writing out the acronym on a piece of paper and filling in each section to reflect each component of your goals. There may be a big picture goal that needs to be broken down into small weekly or bi-weekly goals that will lead up to the big win.

I've seen many people lose sight of their goals because they didn't map a solid plan for how to complete them. I don't want that to be you!

Sometimes all of this strategy and goal setting can feel overwhelming. You may know you want to make some changes in your life but you may not be quite ready to articulate your goals and make a plan. That is okay! There's a way to work through this too.

## When Goal Setting Is Overwhelming

SOMETIME PEOPLE DON'T know what their goals are. I have been met with many blank stares when I have asked new clients to articulate their goals. Some people genuinely feel so stuck that they don't know what they want. Others have lived too long believing they can't have what they dream of; it's almost as if they have forgotten what happiness looks like. When someone can't tell me what their goals are, I ask them the reverse: What do you not want? This usually generates a flood of answers and sometimes even tears. I get a better sense of what they do want through elimination. I was emotionally bankrupt for many years until someone asked me what I didn't want. It turned my ship around.

Kymberly-Nicole is a plus-size athlete and fitness trainer, and she can relate to feeling stuck. Her life was at an all-time low when she decided to find her way back to her athletic roots.

I decided to get into a fitness regime after a very difficult divorce when I was at the lowest point in my life. I was a single mother with a toddler and an infant and no idea what to do next. I slipped into depression and gained more weight than I ever had in my life. I've always been "curvy," but I was at a point where I could barely walk up a flight of stairs. I didn't know what I wanted but I knew that I couldn't live like that anymore. One day I called my mom and said, "I can't do this. I'm no good for my girls; can you please take them for a while?" My mother said yes, of course. However, she told me I wasn't going to be able to keep bringing them to her when things got tough. The girls needed stability, and I needed to make it happen. After swallowing my pride, I made the first of many appointments with a therapist. Through these sessions, I was able to gain clarity by recognizing the things I didn't want in my life. I was able to gain momentum to get back to myself. I had been the captain of my high school cheerleading squad at a size 16. I knew I had the athlete inside of me, and I had to get her back, so each day I started walking, and slowly fitness was a part of my life again! Fitness was a huge part of finding my way back to feeling good about life again and finding my true self.

If you're feeling stuck, think about what you don't want in your life anymore. Keep adding to that list. Over time, you may find that what you do want becomes clearer.

When I was at my lowest, I didn't want to feel crappy about myself anymore, I didn't want to drink anymore, or to feel sick or tired anymore. I wanted new friends. I knew exactly what I didn't want, and it was my starting point for deciphering what

I did want. If this applies to you, make a list of the things you don't want in your life anymore. If you aren't yet ready for SMART goal setting, bookmark this page and return to it later. There will be time for goal setting later.

Because we have been programmed to aspire to narrow cultural ideals, many women believe there is no other goal than to lose weight. They believe their worthiness, and success, is wrapped up in how much they weigh. This is a lie. Worthiness has no size. Women who have tunnel vision with this as a goal generally have the core belief that life will be better if they are thinner, just like I once thought, and that they will be more lovable and more valuable in a thinner body. I ask them to go through a process of identifying what they don't want in order to dig out their hopes and dreams. Sometimes it's things like, "I don't want to feel crappy," or "I don't want to feel so unmotivated"—general feelings of low self-worth. Upon a closer look, it usually has very little to do with weight. People often jump at weight loss when you prompt them to set goals because it's programmed into us that life is bad because you're fat. It may take weeks or months of working with people to demonstrate that health and fitness do not always include weight loss; you can kick ass in the body you have today. Once they start knocking down their fitness goals and building their physical power, I often find that they start to value weight loss less. I model that for them and champion them to get on with their goals in the body they have now. After we work together for some time, many women are able to shift their focus toward fitness-related goals rather than aesthetic aspirations. Often, over time, they will lose some weight as a by-product of working toward those goals but, like me, it's no longer their primary focus.

It is important that we break this cultural spell and learn to rule our own bodies. Our desires and goals need to be our own. This message is starting to be heard by society, but many women still need to relearn what they've been taught and stop waiting to live their dreams. Ask yourself: Are my goals based on my true feelings, or are they shaped by others' expectations of me? Society, family, or others?

Now that you know the stages of change and how to set goals that really create a new lifestyle, how do you make your goals stick?

## Create Positive Thinking

ALL SUCCESSFUL ATHLETES, from everyday warriors to Olympians, share one thing in common: a positive state of mind. One of the simplest yet most powerful principles of sports psychology is the importance of developing positive self-talk. And yet this is one of the hardest skills to master.

Self-love and positive thinking only come through practice. Even if you are unhappy with your body and one of your goals is to lose weight or otherwise change how your body looks, I hope that you feel self-love throughout the journey. Your body now, and at any size, deserves your love and respect. Believing that your body is worthy of love only when it is a certain size will prevent you from accepting yourself and being happy. It will also prevent you from achieving your goals. We can't hate ourselves to a better life; we must be positive and champion ourselves, through every stage, from within.

## Supportive People

EVERY WOMAN DESERVES people who believe in her and support her in everything she wants to accomplish. You need people in your life who believe in your ability, who love you unconditionally, and who stay positive for you even when you aren't feeling so hot.

The relationships we have with our partners, friends, co-workers, and family should be positive and supportive. These people are different from your fitness tribe; they may not understand your crazy desire to get up on a Sunday morning at 7:00 to run in the rain, but they still support you, no matter what. You can't pick your family, but you have a say in how people are allowed to treat you, so be mindful of that and be assertive when needed.

Avoid the people who want to push change on you, who judge your goals according to their own agenda, or who believe they are owed something in return for their support. People who truly care do not make hurtful comments disguised as concern. I've heard clients tell me that their family members make unkind comments followed by, "I'm only concerned for you." I've heard of clients' friends getting annoyed because they are posting too much about how successful and good they feel on social media. These family members and friends are not being supportive. Witnessing these positive changes is clearly triggering for them, and that is one hundred percent their own issue.

Avoid the people who want to hinder your growth, in overt or subtle ways. They may find your success threatening or see your ability to stick to your goals and win as something that is lacking in their own life. Supportive people don't try to talk you out of your workout or encourage you to go out drinking when you have a race the next day. A supportive person joins you at the gym, enjoys that healthy meal with you, or at the very least gives you the space to make your own choices.

Lisa is an avid plus-size athlete who enjoys a range of fitness and adventure activities. She attributes some of her success to the people she surrounds herself with. Lisa's friends work out with her, and her co-workers run with her after work, all because she has expressed her goals and created a circle of people who want to join her in her journey.

Finding the courage to show up was the first step in my shift toward athleticism. But I quickly realized that while showing up is critical, it was only half the battle in claiming athletics as a core part of my life. The second and equally important step was to find my tribe: my supportive people, the ones that believe right along with me (and on occasion, when I don't believe it myself) that I am capable. The population of the tribe changes and evolves all the time for me, but at the root I know that without having my outstanding group of family members, co-workers, and sweat sisters, my athletic pursuits would not be nearly as amazing as they have been.

Rainy nights of run training, learning to box, exploring the awesome discomfort of hot yoga, participating in mud runs, and learning to surf in the chop of the Pacific all required me to show up—yes, but doing them with the group of people I have surrounded myself with has made each endeavor sweeter than the last. There is a bond that forms when you open up and allow people to join you on this journey. And for me the bond with my people has been essential to my success.

As the African proverb says, "If you want to go quickly, go alone. If you want to go farther, go together."

Lisa is a good friend, and she is right. Whether your family and friends join you in your fitness pursuits is up to them, but the people around you need to lift you up, not bring you down.

## Planning

WE'VE ALREADY ESTABLISHED that you need a well-thought-out plan in place. I can't stress this enough. I have been guilty of committing to a race, only to realize once the training begins that I have too much on my plate to properly train. This creates anxiety and takes the joy out of the pursuit. It can also result in being undertrained for an event, and that is never fun, or safe (believe me, don't do it!). Taking time to plan your process in advance sets you up for more success.

Wendy, a fellow plus-size athlete and trainer, plans everything to ensure that she meets her fitness goals. "I do plan out my workouts for the week," she says. "I use my planner and I color-code everything down to my personal plans, my clients, and my workouts so I can see all my commitments in one book. I also have a routine that includes the same times and days because I function much better with routine. It keeps me sane, level-headed and happy."

Planning helps you see how you will get it all done, and it is what lies beneath the success of most finishers at sporting events.

## Accountability

IN CHAPTER THREE, I talked about how fitness buddies or trainers who hold you accountable are essential for long-term commitment to achieving your goals. A group to train with, or a trainer to report to, may help you commit to your new activity. When I first began to run, I needed a running group to keep me committed and focused on my goal of running a 5K. Without this group support, I don't think I would have achieved what I had set out to do. It is possible to achieve your goals alone, but many people need the support of a group to make it happen. When no one expects you to show up, it is easier to just stay home.

## Good Organization

YOU CAN HELP yourself succeed by preparing for your workouts. Pack your gym bag the night before so getting to the gym in the morning is easier. Plan your day so you support your workout time: don't schedule meetings for the end of the day, since a long meeting could cut into your gym time. Prepare your family for your time away—make meals in advance and create routines. Ensuring you are organized and prepared for your workout means you won't be able to say "Screw it, I'm not going." Once workouts become too stressful, they—and your goals—are easily nixed.

## Protect Your Time

I'VE HAD MANY clients tell me they had to work late or a family member needed them so they couldn't make it to class. I see so many women put others first and their own needs second but it's hard to help others when you're not helping yourself first. On airplanes, we've all been told, "Put the oxygen mask on yourself first," which is necessary for survival in an emergency. You need to believe caring for yourself before others is about survival too. I think it's really important to protect your time. If this means approaching your boss to let them know you have commitments on Tuesdays and Thursdays and cannot work late those days, so be it. Employers should support your efforts to be a healthy and happy employee. Remember that bit about supportive people? Employers should be able to offer a healthy balance of life and work, and not drive you into the ground for their own bottom line. Be assertive, boundary-oriented, and protective of your time.

I'VE ALSO WORKED with hundreds of women who let go of dreams to be fit and active because they drive their kids to their activities after work instead. Your kids' lives are enriched by playing sports and having you there to cheer them on, but you offer them a positive role model when you allow yourself time to work hard toward your goals, commit to fitness, and improve your health. Make it a team effort and ask your family to help you schedule time for your own fitness. Some busy moms find early mornings allow them to fit it all in.

Before I had my son, I worked long hours in the film industry. I had one of *those* employers, and I wasn't assertive enough to stand my ground. If I wanted exercise to be a part of my life, I had no choice but to get up at five thirty for a boot camp class that began at six o'clock. At my job, getting away at lunchtime wasn't likely, so early mornings it was or fitness went out the window. At first it was difficult to get up early, but I got used to it and then realized that early morning exercise helped me start my day with fantastic energy. I highly recommend it if it works with your schedule!

If you falter in protecting your time, you send out a message that this time is negotiable. Putting your health and well-being first shouldn't be open for negotiation—be that CEO! In my program, I've seen many women who feel guilty taking time for themselves. There's no place for guilt here; you are worth the care and attention, and when you are taken care of you have the energy to care for others. But you come first.

Living like an athlete requires setting solid boundaries and adds an extra layer of planning and organization to your life. It will become easier with practice, and your commitment will become more solid as you experience the positive effects of exercise. Exercise has become my lifeline. The new me needs exercise to function in everyday life. I have found joy, empowerment, friends, and a positive state of mind that helps me be a better parent, wife, community member, and business owner. I have done it all by being SMART, one goal at a time.

# SIX

# Peace, Love, and Food

FOOD IS A sensitive topic for many people. Relationships with food can be complex and they are shaped when we are very young. I vividly remember, at four or five years old, asking my dad for a snack one afternoon. He responded, "You always want to eat when you are bored." That is the first time I remember feeling ashamed for wanting food.

Although my dad's words made me feel bad, he was right. Even at that young age I was using food for more than just nourishment. Food was a form of entertainment; I ate because I was bored or because I was feeling lonely. As time went on, I used food to heal emotional wounds and ate to manage stress and anxiety. To be honest, there are still days when I use food for more than nourishment.

As I got older, I tried to manage my eating habits and weight through dieting. I found myself in the loop of restrictive eating, followed by binge eating, followed by restrictive eating. This way of eating never felt good. The food I chose was making me sick, literally, and I developed food sensitivities and a pervasive feeling of fatigue. Back then I ate a lot of deep-fried

Chinese food, pizza as a regular staple, and most mornings I ate baked goods, and I felt tired all the time. I had headaches and recurring acne, and my motivation to do anything was at an all-time low. I would flip from pizza mode to salad mode and then back into eating whatever the hell I wanted. I didn't have any concept of what healthy eating was.

We live in a culture that sends mixed messages about food. We are constantly bombarded with advertising for big juicy hamburgers you can barely get your mouth around or pizza lifted out of the box with the cheese stretching invitingly across the television screen. I recently learned that tactic of stretching cheese is referred to as "cheese pull" and is used in advertising to entice you to dial up and order.

The cheese pull is more than just a tantalizing glimpse of melted goodness. Advertisers use it to communicate with the part of our brain that's not verbal, the primal core of our being that doesn't understand words but responds with hunger, thirst, arousal, desire. Advertisers and food corporations are subconsciously priming us to want their food. But while one commercial might feature cheese pulling, the next could be for a diet product, creating mixed messages about what we should eat.

Food is about more than just survival. Food is social. It is part of our celebrations: birthdays, Christmas, Thanksgiving, weddings, and other occasions often center around lots of food. Food is as often a reward as it is sustenance. Food also plays a role in depression, coping, and sometimes punishing ourselves through binge eating or through deprivation. It can be nourishing and a source of cultural pride, but it also has the ability to isolate and to control. Food controls many women as they pursue a perfectionist ideal, and food controlled my life for many years. When I gave up dieting, I also gave up a cluttered mind full of chatter around food. What I would eat that day, what I could eat if I exercised for an hour. If I met my friends for dinner, would I blow it? How many calories were in that dish? A constant mental monologue about food that dominated my thoughts.

Food and our complex reactions to it take up mental space, but it remains essential to human survival. We need food to live. If you struggle with eating, the necessity of food is the biggest challenge because you cannot abstain from food like you can with cigarettes, alcohol, or drugs. In order to live healthfully, we must learn to manage this ever-so-complex relationship with food.

The food industry is driven by capitalism. Health is often overlooked in favor of commerce. Fast-food restaurants and pre-packaged convenience foods do not contribute to our health and well-being but instead encourage us to quickly consume great amounts of food, leading to more and more profit for manufacturers whose only concern is the bottom line. To maximize profits on nutritionally empty foods, advertisers come at us with promises and solutions: it's easy, it's quick, it's delicious, and millions of people are buying in.

The food industry and the diet industry are closely related: they both bombard us with tantalizing but empty promises. It can be a challenge to keep up with the latest diet trends— from low fat to low carb to bacon at every meal. How are we supposed to know what is good for us? The possibilities are overwhelming.

## End the Struggle with Food

I BECAME SERIOUS about my health in my late twenties when I first took up running. It was several years later, however, that I started to work toward a better relationship with food. I thought I was doing a good job; now I realize I was in a chronic cycle of dieting, and it was harming rather than help-ing my body.

As I reached my thirties I started to consider my family his-tory. My grandmother died of a stroke in her early fifties, as did two of her siblings. My dad was diagnosed with high blood pressure before he was forty. He went to the doctor for severe chronic headaches, and his blood pressure was so high in his first reading that his doctor immediately sent him to the emer-gency room. Through my genetics, I know I am susceptible to certain health conditions; my dad jokes that our family is cursed. But it's not a joke; I take these predispositions seriously so I can enjoy my life with my husband and son for as long as I can.

Regular exercise helped me learn to view food not as the enemy but as something that could propel me further into ath-letic success. I started eating healthy, nutrient-dense foods to protect myself from my health predispositions; sometimes I do this well and sometimes not. But I no longer view food as "good" or "bad." I am a work in progress. I no longer deprive myself for the sake of attaining some ideal body shape, but rather eat healthfully to live longer and better.

Today I enjoy all foods in moderation—salads, grains, meats, and sometimes pizza and ice cream—and in this way I am able to achieve a healthy, vibrant balance rather than constantly restricting and compensating by eating foods that made me feel unwell.

If you relate to my story, ask yourself whether your relation-ship with food needs to be improved. The truth is, the primary purpose of eating food is survival. As you become more active, your body will demand more nutrient-dense food and you will likely crave healthy foods. Exercise can make you really hun-gry; honor that and give your body what it needs.

With more activity you will likely become hungrier, and if you replenish your body with empty calories such as baked

goods made with white flour and sugars or other empty carbohydrates, you will find that you are always hungry and your
physical performance will suffer.

And as you bring healthier foods into your life, you will start
to crave these foods more and more. Don't push this evolution;
let it flow from this initial step. Let go of your battle with food
and start eating like an athlete with abundant nutrition. Hunger shouldn't be a part of your health plan. What if you just ate
for nourishment? Now is a good time for imagery and visualization. Think about it.

**Amanda Trusty, body-positive blogger, dancer, teacher:**
"I'm really exploring what healthy means to me. I'm a little over
two years into eating disorder recovery, and I am at a place
where I really don't have fear around food, which is what I consider
my biggest victory. I've decided the only way to manage eating
without craziness for the rest of my life is to adopt a model of
abundance over restriction, adding healthy foods rather than
taking foods away."

## Non-Restrictive Approach to Eating

A NON-RESTRICTIVE APPROACH to eating encourages you
to embrace your body today. It takes you away from the diet
mentality; the choices you make in the kitchen are not about
changing the way you look, because you are amazing already.
They are about changing the way you feel. As you start to use
high-quality fuel, you will begin to feel better, and the rewards
will motivate you to keep going. This approach to eating frees
you from the immense pressure to become someone else and
rids your mind of incessant chatter about food. This mental

clarity will propel you closer to your athletic dreams. Non-restrictive eating has allowed me to accept the person I am and the body I live in and freed me from the vicious cycle of try and fail, over and over again. It released me from diminishing self-esteem that came with every failure when I realized I couldn't adhere to the demands of diets. I know what my body needs; yours might be different. The key is that there's no "good" or "bad" language about food. You should be able to enjoy all foods in a healthful way.

My relationship with food is a continuous exploration. I keep learning what works for me. As I become more aware of my behavior around food, I gain healthy insight that allows me to repair that broken relationship. I still want to eat when I feel anxious or bored, but I now have an awareness that helps me rethink using food for coping. I have had the privilege to learn from others in my tribe, including many who are changing the diet paradigm from "get thin" to "get healthy."

## How to Make Peace with Food

BE NOURISHED IS a revolutionary business that offers a curriculum of health teaching that leads participants away from disordered eating patterns toward radical self-care and healing. Co-founders Hilary Kinavey, a registered counselor, and Dana Sturtevant, a registered dietitian, pursue a mission to help people heal body dissatisfaction and reclaim trust in their own bodies, a process they refer to as building "body trust." Here are their recommendations to help you heal body shame, make peace with food, and create the change you seek from a deeper place.

Understanding (and healing) your relationship with food is less about doing it right and more about learning ways to take care of yourself that are enjoyable and sustainable. When we try to "fix" our bodies or pursue weight loss, we often end up making most of our decisions from our head, completely cut off from our bodies. Our dieting culture is mistrustful of bodies and is pretty obsessed with "doing the right thing" all of the time, which comes at a great cost.

Can you imagine choosing to eat for your body instead of trying to follow the constantly changing rules of the dieting mind? Eating the "right" way can leave you feeling deficient in satisfaction and pleasure. Eating from your head, without consulting your body, leads to great disconnection from the intelligence of your hungers and appetites. Eating in attunement with your body returns you to your innate wisdom, making you feel at peace with your food choices again. We invite awareness, not perfection, and see each eating experience as an opportunity to learn and practice.

Your relationship with food and your body has been a way of coping. When you are able to understand that that personal struggle is part of the experience of being human, you are more able to speak your truth, move away from shame, and act in the interest of your own well-being. When you have compassion and empathy for others, you feel warmth, caring and act kindly toward them. The same can happen when you increase compassion for yourself. It is in this space of acceptance that the capacity for change increases, and your relationship to your body and your self begins to feel different. No longer will you have to measure your worth and your progress by the number on the scale or the size of your jeans. Discover more meaningful markers of your health and wellness: reduced body hatred, increased trust with food, more satisfaction and joy in your life and feeling more confident in your own skin. Imagine that!

Hilary and Dana are doing amazing food-related work with their clients. You can find more resources at benourished.com.

## The Underbelly of the Issues

MANY FITNESS BOOKS prescribe how to get fit and lose weight without discussing issues such as emotional and addictive eating, which is like slapping a Band-Aid on a wound without investigating the cause of the wound.

Christy is a plus-size athlete from Vancouver. Growing up in a dysfunctional home, she learned to use food as a coping mechanism.

As a kid, if it wasn't mac and cheese, hot dogs, takeout, or from a bag, I didn't eat it. Not because I was a picky eater, but because as a child that was the only way I could feed myself because my parents were alcoholics and drug addicts. Their priorities did not consist of teaching me about food or nutrition. Instead, the focus was on keeping my little brother and me occupied. Initially, I ate food that was easy to prepare; then I turned to food for boredom and then I'd turn to food to change my feelings. I often felt that my family didn't love me, that I was different from my friends, and that I needed to hide the way our family lived. Once I learned that food could change the way I felt, there was no turning back.

I would use food to stuff down the feelings I had about my abusive childhood. As I grew older, I would use food to ignore my feelings about being bullied and humiliated. And as an adult, I would use food to manage my stress levels from the high standards I placed on myself to make my adult life better than my childhood.

It wasn't until I was faced with years of infertility due to polycystic ovary syndrome that I had to take my relationship with food seriously. I was thirty years old when I had to learn that food was fuel and that I needed to learn to cope with emotions with skill instead of substances—and in my case it was sugar. My parents may have abused drugs and alcohol but I was abusing food. It took dedicated classes learning about nutrition and portions, meetings with nutritionists, and a complete revolution around eating to confront my relationship with food and the control I gave it over my feelings. I am proud to say that I make my decisions with an educated perspective instead of impulsively with my emotions now.

Christy's story is a familiar one. Maybe her circumstances are not the same as yours or mine, but her story of how she used food for reasons other than nutrition may be similar. Fixing the problem is not as simple as saying "just stop eating that." Recognize that this part of your journey may not be an easy one. Start with the principles mentioned above, to build body trust, and then introduce some of these strategies for adopting healthier food habits.

## Healthier Food Habits

### SWITCHING OUT FOODS

When I eliminate a type of food from my diet, it isn't because it is high in calories or fat. I switch it out because it just isn't right for me: it makes me feel tired or unwell or leads to incessant cravings. Sugar is a big one for me. When I eat sugar regularly, it leads to wanting it more and more, so although sugar is still part of my nutrition, I try to limit it. This is a different mindset from dieting, which labels food "good" or "bad" and makes you believe everyone should avoid the bad. Switching out foods is replacing them with different foods—not reducing or restricting. It is also different from dieting.

It is possible to replace foods that don't make you feel good with similar foods that do. For example, instead of takeout pizza, try homemade pizza, with a quality whole-grain crust and fresh vegetables as toppings. Takeout pizza is often filled with low-quality sodium-packed cheese, which can leave you feeling thirsty and bloated. Your homemade pizza is less likely to give you that feeling.

**PREPARE YOUR MEALS**

It's hard to know exactly what you are consuming if you eat out a lot. But it is well known that much restaurant food is high in sodium. When I eat foods high in sodium, my eyelids get very puffy, I'm chronically thirsty, and I just don't feel well. The Mayo Clinic reports that optimal sodium intake should be at a maximum of 2,300 mg per day; yet, according to the Mayo Clinic the average American consumes closer to 3,400 mg per day.[1] I don't want to engage in fear mongering—I know this because of my own family history, and studies show that chronic high sodium intake can lead to high blood pressure and heart disease. When you prepare your food at home, you can control the amount of sodium you take in. And when you avoid prepackaged food, you generally reduce your sodium to include only the forms found naturally in food.

I try to limit eating out to two or three times a month, not only because of the expense and how it sometimes makes me feel, but also because high sodium isn't good for me, especially given my family history. Here are some suggestions from the Heart and Stroke Foundation on how to avoid high levels of sodium intake for your optimal health and for your best athletic performance.[2] These tips should give you some ideas for feeling great.

- Eat mostly fresh foods prepared at home and eat fewer ready-made packaged foods.

- Develop and share food preparation and cooking skills.
- Limit eating at restaurants and fast-food outlets, ask for nutrition information, and ask for meals to be prepared with no salt when dining out.
- Reduce the amount of salt used in cooking by not adding the full amount a recipe calls for.
- Wash away some of the salt in canned goods such as beans, lentils, and vegetables by rinsing them before eating.
- Cut down on the amount of seasoning used when making packaged pastas or taco kits.
- Taste food before adding salt. Add salt-free herbs and spices or lemon to foods for extra flavor instead of salt.
- Look for "sodium-free," "low sodium," "reduced sodium," or "no added salt" on the package if choosing packaged foods.

## PORTIONS

If you are like me and have been a chronic dieter, you know all about portion control. These days, I never worry about portions; I eat until I am satisfied. Depending on my workout schedule, this can be a huge amount of food (seriously, sometimes I feel like I have a hollow leg) or not much at all. You should pay attention to portions not to restrict calories but to maintain your energy levels. When I eat too much, I just want to lie down and sleep, and that does not help me to reach my goals. I urge you to manage your portions as a way to manage your energy for athletic performance. It also helps to practice mindful eating, which means to eat with intention while paying attention. This can be done by chewing slowly, turning off the phone and television and other distractions, paying attention to the flavors as you chew, and listening carefully to your body's cues that you are sated. Mindful eating is a practice used to avoid its opposite, mindless eating while on the run, in the car, or at your work desk while not really experiencing the ritual of nourishing your body.

## AVOID GETTING HANGRY

"Hangry" is a slang term for that angry feeling that results from hunger. I get very hangry when I've waited too long between meals and allowed my blood sugar to drop too much. Once my blood sugar is low, I start to get tired and irritable, and I lose concentration. Then, in this mindless state, I get tunnel vision and go on a mission to eat anything and everything in sight. It never ends well. I usually find myself slumped on the couch, exhausted, and this does *nothing* for athletic performance! A good rule of thumb is to eat every three hours. It doesn't have to be a big meal, but have snacks on hand to avoid plummeting blood sugar and hangry binge eating. In a state of hanger, working out isn't a good idea; you need nourishing food to perform, always.

## EAT FOR ATHLETIC PERFORMANCE

As you become more active, you may find that you want to eat more; athletes eat a lot of food! To support the hard work you put in at the gym, pool, or track, you will need fuel to supply your muscles with the energy they need to perform. What you eat should fuel your athletic pursuits, and that means an abundance of healthy, energy-rich foods. This is not a model of restriction; I'm sure you're happy to hear that!

Sarah Robles is a two-time Olympic athlete who eats to perform well. For her, this means eating simply:

> Generally speaking, I'm not too strict. If I'm not gaining or losing too much weight too fast and I can recover from training and I have the energy to complete my training, then I am happy. I'm a fan of sticking to the basics—adhering to a well-rounded diet with lean meats, fruits and vegetables, and whole grains. Eat with a purpose and remember you are a machine. Every person has different needs, but the core needs are still there to fuel your body with nutritionally dense foods.

HERE ARE SOME ideas to feed your athletic performance.

## Nourishing Pre-Workout

IT'S IMPORTANT TO avoid exercising on a full stomach. Food that remains in your stomach during exercise may cause nausea and cramping. To make sure you have enough energy, yet to reduce stomach discomfort, you should allow a meal to fully digest before you work out. This generally takes anywhere from one to two hours, depending on how much you have eaten. Everyone is different, and you should experiment with what works for you before a workout to determine your ideal eating schedule.

If you have an early morning race or workout, get up early enough to eat a pre-exercise meal or snack. Consume something that digests quickly, like a smoothie. However, it's really important to find out what works for you and your body. A smoothie isn't going to work for everyone, and finding your go-to pre-workout meal can be done by exploring what you like with a trial-and-error approach to discover what makes you feel the most energized.

Before you head out for a workout, it's important to make sure your body is hydrated. Dehydration will leave you feeling lethargic and may cause headaches or poor performance and even predispose you to injury. Taking water to the gym or on your run is good, but it isn't enough; consume water throughout the day to help your body function at its top level while you are exercising.

Your pre-workout meal or snack should include quality carbs, protein, and heart-healthy fats. Your muscles rely on carbohydrate foods like breads, cereals, pasta, rice, fruits, and vegetables for quick energy and protein for building and repair.

Avoid refined sugars throughout your training period. Refined sugar is found in cakes, candy, syrups, ready-to-eat cereals, flavored yogurt, and many other processed foods. Refined sugars are absorbed quickly into the bloodstream and can cause a spike in blood sugar. To perform well athletically, and to feel good in daily life, try to keep your blood sugar level by eating regularly and avoiding foods high in sugar. I admit that I really enjoy some sugary foods, so if I am going to indulge I make sure it is after my training is done.

If you are hitting the gym after work, have a light snack like an apple and some almonds. It's best to fuel up for your workout with energy that will manage your blood sugar to avoid crashes and cravings. Eating an apple along with some protein, like almonds, helps manage the sugar that enters your blood stream from the apple. It's always a good idea to couple carbohydrates (or sugars) with proteins to avoid spikes that inevitably cause crashes resulting in tiredness. Remember, peak performance and energy levels are the goal.

Here are some great ideas for small pre-workout meals that include quality carbohydrates and protein:

- Natural peanut butter and whole-grain toast
- Natural Greek yogurt and fruit
- Almonds and an apple
- A banana–Greek yogurt smoothie
- Chicken, rice, and vegetables
- Tofu, quinoa, and vegetables
- Hummus, vegetables, and whole-wheat crackers
- Oatmeal, fruit, and plain Greek yogurt
- Oatmeal, nuts, and plain Greek yogurt
- Hardboiled egg and carrot and celery sticks

## Nourishing Post-Workout

DURING YOUR WORKOUT your body uses the glycogen stores in your muscles as fuel. Glycogen is a substance deposited in body tissues as a store of carbohydrates; it is what gives you the energy to perform well in fitness. You have probably experienced a workout when you felt you just didn't have it in you. One cause could be low glycogen stores from inadequate fueling. Glycogen acts like money in a bank. You can't just top it up with a pre-workout meal right before a workout; you need to make regular deposits and avoid withdrawing more than you have. Eat throughout the day to maintain a healthy level of blood sugar, manage hunger, and keep your energy stores topped up.

Post-workout meals and snacks should include protein for muscle repair. Have you ever had a workout where you've been sore for days afterward? It could be for a number of reasons, but one of them might be insufficient nutrition to repair your muscles quickly. Sound nutrition, with optimal portions of protein, is a must for repairing muscles post-workout. Muscle protein breaks down during exercise and undergoes repair during post-workout recovery. Between workouts your muscles are synthesizing new fibers, and this process is aided by your protein intake. To meet your body's needs for muscle building and repair, you should consume protein fairly quickly after your workout.

How much protein you need after a training session is linked to how much protein you consume daily. The USDA recommended daily intake of protein is 0.66 grams of protein per two pounds of body weight. However, anyone undergoing intense training should consume slightly more protein, somewhere around 1 to 1.8 grams per 2.2 pounds of body weight.[3] It's also a good idea to split your protein intake between all of your meals, so post-workout snacks should include a portion of that protein.

Here are some ideas for protein-based post-workout snacks or meals to aid in muscle restoration.

· Trail mix
· Protein smoothie
· Scrambled eggs and toast
· Tuna sandwich
· Turkey wraps
· Protein bar (be careful here; many have lots of sugar, which can make you tired)

THE FOLLOWING FOODS are good building blocks for nutrient-dense meals and snacks that support your athletic way of life. The possible combinations are endless and delicious.

## Protein

Beans: *Chickpeas, kidney beans, black beans, lentils, butter beans, baked beans, soya beans*
White fish: *Cod, halibut, haddock, sole, pollock*
Oily fish: *Salmon, sardines, mackerel, fresh tuna, trout*
Shellfish: *Prawns, scallops, mussels, oysters, squid, crab*
Poultry: *Chicken, turkey*
Eggs
Other sources of protein: *Nuts, nut milks, peanut butter, tofu, soy milks, whey*

## Complex Carbohydrates

Vegetables: *Potatoes, sweet potatoes, yams, squash, onions, dill pickles, carrots, radishes, broccoli, spinach, green beans, zucchini, cucumbers, asparagus*

Fruits: *Grapefruit, apples, pears, prunes, strawberries, melons, apples, oranges*

Grains: *Brown rice, wild rice, couscous, barley, quinoa, oatmeal, corn*

Beans and legumes: *Black beans, kidney beans, lentils, peas*

Breads, pastas, and cereals: *Whole-wheat bread, high-fiber cereal, whole-wheat tortillas, whole-wheat pita bread, whole grains, whole-wheat pasta*

AND DON'T FORGET about healthy fats. Diet culture has given this brainfood a bad rap. Fat doesn't necessarily make you fat. And you need the nutrients in fatty foods for healthy brain function, a healthy heart, and peak athletic performance.

## Healthy Fats

Nuts: *Almonds, walnuts, cashews, pecans, hazelnuts*

Nut butter: *Almond butter, peanut butter, cashew butter, hazelnut butter*

Milks: *Almond milk, coconut milk, soy milk*

Seeds: *Flax, hemp, sunflower, pumpkin, chia, sesame seeds*

Oils: *Olive oil, canola oil, sesame oil, coconut oil*

Vegetables and fruits: *Avocados, olives*

Fish: *Salmon, trout, halibut, sardines*

Tofu

THE FOODS LISTED here contain no added sugars, salt, or preservatives and are nutritionally dense enough for your highest athletic achievements.

## Not All Healthy-Looking Food Is Healthy!

IF YOU FIND yourself in the health food aisle looking at snack options, be careful. Sometimes food that looks or sounds "healthy" really isn't. Don't be fooled by clever marketing, buzzwords, and phrases such as "contains no trans fats" and "gluten free." People often equate "organic" with "healthy." But organic potato chips are still potato chips. If you are unsure whether a food is good for you or not, read the label. If it contains ingredients that you can't pronounce, it might be a good idea to pass on it. Better yet, reach for food that has no label at all. Processed food contains added sugar and salt, ingredients that are not conducive to optimal athletic performance.

As well, many food companies will try to hide "sugar" under a different name. Watch out for these ingredients.

**OTHER NAMES FOR SUGAR:**

| | |
|---|---|
| barley malt | glucose |
| beet sugar | glucose solids |
| brown sugar | golden sugar |
| buttered syrup | golden syrup |
| cane juice crystals | grape sugar |
| cane sugar | honey |
| caramel | invert sugar |
| carob syrup | lactose |
| corn syrup | maltodextrin |
| corn syrup solids | maltose |
| date sugar | mannitol |
| dextran | molasses |
| dextrose | raw sugar |
| diastase | refiner's syrup |
| diastatic malt | sorbitol |
| ethyl maltol | sorghum syrup |
| fructose | sucrose |
| fruit juice | turbinado sugar |
| fruit juice concentrate | yellow sugar |

## The Exercise Reward Trap

I HAVE BEEN guilty of rewarding myself with food after a difficult training session. I may justify my actions by saying to myself: "I worked out, so I can eat whatever I want." And sometimes I've been guilty of taking that mindset too far, sabotaging my great post-workout feelings.

How I start my day with food generally sets the tone for the rest of the day, so if I go for a long run and then follow it up with a big pancake breakfast, that could lead to more empty carbohydrates throughout the day. Running can make you extremely hungry, but if you replenish your body with empty calories, chances are you'll keep going for more and more empty calories because your body is never really getting the replenishment it needs. The end result is that you eat all day and you're never satisfied.

Planning your post-workout meals is essential because after your workout, in a tired and hangry state, your defenses might be down and you may ravenously eat anything in sight. Remember, you are trying to optimize your energy levels post-workout and store that energy for your next workout. If you haven't planned your meals and there's food you want to eat, ask yourself: Does this fuel my next training session? I try to listen to my body and give it what it needs for optimal functioning—both inside the gym and in my daily life. Working out and eating do not have a "tit for tat" relationship. And exercise itself is the real reward! If you find yourself regularly wanting to pat yourself on the back with big meals and treats, find a reward that is not associated with food. A massage or pedicure after a difficult run are great ways to reward yourself. We all like some pampering.

Associating food with "reward" is often a habit learned in childhood, when adults might say "Good job" while offering a treat. Try to find other rewards that can be even more satisfying. For example, buy something you can use when you work out, such as a new water bottle or headband; enter your next event as a reward; take the afternoon for yourself and swing in a hammock or read a book; or buy yourself some flowers.

Changing the way you view food is a noble but difficult battle. But it becomes easier with every change you make. Like me, you may be fighting habits that have been ingrained in you by childhood experiences and by our culture. In our adult lives, we are told to restrict calories but at the same time are bombarded with temptations of food all around us. Food manufacturers want us to become hooked on their cheezies and mini-muffins. It is up to you to break from those habits and pay attention to what your body wants and needs to be the best athlete you can.

Here are eight tips I have found transformative that have improved my relationship with food and kicked my athleticism up a notch. See if they work for you too.

1. Smash the scale. I stopped using a scale as a measure of my health and now listen to and look at other cues from my body.
2. Focus on the "why" rather than the "what." I pay attention to why I eat rather than what I eat.
3. Eat mindfully. I continue to work on eating only when I am hungry. I practice staying connected to my body by being present at meal times, ensuring I have few distractions.
4. Find your motivation. When my son was born, I became extra motivated because not only do I want to be here for him as long as I can, but I also want to model a healthy lifestyle for him.
5. Abandon restrictive eating and adopt an athlete's habit of consuming abundant, healthy, performance-enhancing

nutrition. I now focus on eating healthfully for life and athletic performance. This has been the biggest shift for me, and it has helped me pay attention to what my body needs and wants.

6. Reduce refined sugars. This is a personal choice for me because I need to manage my blood sugar levels, and because I feel crazy around sugar. I have the most energy for my busy life when I limit my intake of refined sugars to an occasional treat.

7. Practice body love. I practice body love often by overriding any negative inner dialogue and giving my body what it needs: exercise, sleep, quiet time, and good nutrition. When I love my body, I want the best for it and that translates into healthy practices with both food and exercise.

8. If you decide to work with a dietician or nutritionist, interview them to see if they work from a weight-neutral approach. Through nutrition, I pursue my goals of elevating my athleticism and health, and I have surrounded myself with professionals who understand this approach.

NONE OF THIS is about policing your food; it's about being your healthiest, most athletic self and finding freedom from being controlled by food and the negative emotional power it may carry. Every body deserves peace and love around food, but it will take some work to get there! Are you ready?

# Big Fit Girl
# Recipe Vault

As we've discussed, one of my struggles has been to shed the diet mentality. You know what I mean—eating ultra-low-fat cream cheese, tuna with no mayo, and plain rice crackers (which is like eating air), not to mention the constant mental tracking, all while feeling hungry. I was unhappy and on edge most of the time. I eventually stopped weighing and measuring my food and counting calories and started eating foods that were nutritionally dense and that increased my energy and enhanced my athletic performance. These steps greatly improved my life.

I am always working on my relationship with food, and I've realized that there is no "perfect" way to eat. You have to do what feels right for your body, and that may be different from what feels right to someone else.

To say that I love food is an understatement. I simply can't live without great-tasting, satisfying meals. My days of living in hunger are over, and they can be over for you too. Here are some of the recipes that work for me and that I hope might work for you.

## Breakfast

### GREEN GURU SMOOTHIE FROM BUDDHA-FULL.CA

6 oz. apple juice
$^1/_2$ cup mango, cut up
$^1/_2$ cup pineapple, cut up
1 cup spinach leaves
3 pitted dates
$^1/_2$ cup ice

Blend in a blender until smooth.

## LOBO SMOOTHIE FROM BUDDHA-FULL.CA

6 oz. almond milk

2 bananas

3 oz. smooth peanut butter

4 pitted dates

1 tbsp. hemp protein (high density)

$\frac{1}{2}$ cup ice

Blend in a blender until smooth.

## OVERNIGHT BLUEBERRY-CINNAMON OATS

$\frac{1}{2}$ cup rolled oats

$\frac{1}{2}$ cup almond, soy, or cow's milk

$\frac{1}{2}$ tsp. cinnamon, more or less, to preference

$\frac{1}{2}$ cup frozen blueberries

Add all ingredients to a Mason jar, seal, and refrigerate. Let soak overnight.

Variations can be made by adding strawberries, raspberries, or other fruit to your liking.

## BREAKFAST BANANA CHOCOLATE CHIP COOKIES
### FROM AMANDA LEITH

$2\frac{1}{3}$ cups quick oats

$\frac{3}{4}$ tsp. salt

1 tsp. ground cinnamon

1 cup almond butter

$\frac{1}{4}$ cup pure maple syrup

2 large, ripe bananas, mashed (about 1 cup)

$\frac{1}{3}$ cup dark or semi-sweet cocolate chips and/or raisins

$\frac{1}{3}$ cup sliced almonds

Preheat oven to 325ºF. Line a large baking sheet with parchment paper.

Combine all ingredients until thoroughly mixed. The dough will be sticky and thick.

Use 3 tbsp. dough for each cookie. Drop dough onto prepared baking sheet and slightly flatten the tops into desired thickness. The cookies will not spread in the oven. Bake for 15 minutes, until edges are very slightly brown. Don't bake any longer or the cookies will taste dry. Cool and serve.

## Lunch

### MEXICAN RICE BOWL

### Bowl

$1/2$ cup cooked brown rice
$1/2$ cup rinsed black beans
$1/2$ avocado
$1/2$ cup cooked corn
Canned or fresh salsa, a little or a lot, to your preference
1 oz. shredded cheddar cheese
2 tsp. chopped cilantro
$1/2$ cup shredded red cabbage

Arrange all the ingredients in a bowl.

### Light Dressing

*Note: There is a ton of flavor in this bowl so use dressing sparingly. Refrigerate remainder for your next bowl.*
Juice of 1 lime
1 tsp. clear honey
1 tsp. chili powder
3 tbsp. olive oil

Mix with a blender or whisk. Add desired amount of dressing to your bowl when you are ready to eat.

## FREESTYLE FRITTATA

8 large eggs

1/4 cup milk

1/2 tsp. salt

3/4 tsp. pepper

Add whatever else you've got in the fridge. Here are some ideas:

Spinach, tomato, feta

Zucchini, mushroom, peppers, cheese

Ham, cheese, rosemary

Freestyle it to your preference!

Bake in an oven-safe skillet at 350°F for 15 minutes or until egg pulls away from edges. Let cool for 10 minutes and serve. Great the next day: bring it to work and heat it up, add some veggies or salad to the side. This meal packs a lot of protein punch!

## Salads

## STRAWBERRY, FETA, SPINACH SALAD

### Salad

3 cups torn spinach leaves

1 cup arugula

8 cherry or grape tomatoes sliced in half or whole

5–10 chopped strawberries (depending on preference)

1/2 avocado

1/4 cup toasted walnuts

1 tbsp. crumbled feta cheese

Combine all ingredients in a salad bowl.

### Dressing

2 cloves garlic

1 tbsp. pure maple syrup

¼ cup red wine vinegar

1 tbsp. grainy mustard

1 tbsp. balsamic vinegar

¾ cup fresh basil leaves

Salt and pepper to taste

¾ cup olive oil

Blend all ingredients in a blender or food processor. Cover and set aside.

Right before serving pour desired amount of dressing over salad. Lightly toss and serve.

### SPINACH SALAD WITH CURRY & CHUTNEY DRESSING
FROM AMANDA LEITH

#### Salad

4 cups spinach torn into bite-size pieces

1½ cups tart apple, coarsely chopped

½ cup chopped green onion

1 cup dry roasted peanuts

Combine all ingredients in a salad bowl.

#### Dressing

¼ cup apple cider or red wine vinegar

¼ cup olive oil

3 tbsp. mango chutney

1½ tsp. curry powder

⅛ tsp. turmeric

Pinch of salt

Blend all ingredients in a blender or food processor. Cover and set aside.

Right before serving pour desired amount of dressing over salad. Lightly toss and serve.

## SMOKED GRUYERE CABBAGE SALAD
FROM AMANDA LEITH

### Salad

1 cup diced red pepper

1 cup diced long English cucumber

1 cup finely chopped snap peas

1 cup finely chopped green cabbage

1 cup finely chopped purple cabbage

1 cup diced smoked Gruyere cheese

1 cup whole unsalted raw almonds

Roast almonds in 350°F oven for approximately 10 minutes; watch closely, as nuts can burn quickly. When finished let cool. Chop all other ingredients and combine. When almonds are cool enough, chop and add to salad.

### Dressing

$1/4$ cup apple cider vinegar

$1/2$ cup olive oil

1 tsp. honey Dijon mustard

1 tsp. honey (optional)

2 cloves finely chopped garlic

Salt and pepper

Combine all ingredients in a glass jar with lid. Shake vigorously until well combined. Dress salad and toss.

## Dinner

### SHRIMP TACOS FROM SUPERYOU.CA

4 large brown rice or whole-grain tortillas

Frozen cooked shrimp (about $1 1/4$ cups per person; they shrink when they cook)

1 lime for juicing
1 tsp. avocado oil or olive oil
1 tsp. chili powder
Salt to taste

Cook shrimp in a non-stick skillet with a lid. Once the shrimp has begun to sauté, squeeze in 1/2 lime and oil. After a minute of sautéing, add chili powder and pinch of salt. As the shrimp cooks, make the slaw and warm the tortillas.

### Slaw

1/4 red cabbage, chopped fine
1 red or yellow pepper, chopped fine
2 green onions, chopped fine
1 tbsp. apple cider vinegar
1 tbsp. avocado olive or olive oil
Salt and pepper to taste

Combine all ingredients in a bowl.
Layer slaw on top of warmed tortillas and top with the shrimp.

### IRISH STEW

2 1/2 lbs. beef chuck
2 coarsely chopped onions
4 cloves garlic
1/2 tsp. coarse black pepper
1/4 tsp. sea salt
1 tbsp. fresh rosemary
1 cup water or 1/2 can Guinness (your preference)
1/4 cup tomato paste
3 carrots, chopped in rounds
2 celery stalks, chopped
2 1/2 cups beef stock (or as needed to cover)
Cornstarch (as needed for desired thickness)

Brown the beef in a large stewing pot, about 3 minutes per side on medium-high. Once the meat is brown, slowly add onions, garlic, salt, pepper, and rosemary. After a few minutes add water or Guinness and let simmer for 2–3 minutes. Add tomato paste and beef stock and bring to a boil; boil for 2–3 minutes. Add remaining vegetable ingredients and simmer for 2 hours, stirring occasionally. Add a teaspoon (or more, as needed) of cornstarch to bring to desired thickness.

Optional: Serve over mashed potatoes.

## SALMON BURGER WITH PESTO MAYO

### Salmon

4 oz. salmon fillets, skinned and boned
1 tbsp. vegetable oil or canola oil
Lemon juice from 2 lemons
1 clove garlic, finely chopped

Combine oil, lemon juice, and garlic and brush on salmon fillets. Pan-fry for 3–4 minutes per side on medium-high heat.

### Pesto Mayo

1 oz. basil
1/2 garlic glove
Dash salt and pepper
3 tbsp. olive oil
2 tbsp. mayo

Dress your favorite buns with pesto mayo, butter lettuce, red onion, and tomato. Add salmon patty. Serve with your choice of salad.

## Sweets

### APPLE PEAR CRUMBLE FROM SUPERYOU.CA

2 pears, peeled and chopped
2 apples, peeled and chopped
1 tbsp. melted coconut oil
$1/2$ cup large-flake oats
2 tbsp. brown sugar
2 tsp. cinnamon

Place apples and pears in a bake-safe dish and sprinkle with 1 tsp. cinnamon. Mix to spread the cinnamon. In a small dish mix the oats, coconut oil, brown sugar, and remaining 1 tsp. cinnamon. Sprinkle over the fruit mixture. Bake at 425°F for about 20 minutes. Let sit for 5-10 minutes to cool before serving.

### BLUEBERRY LEMON FLAN

#### Crust

1 cup whole-wheat flour
$1/4$ cup brown sugar
$1/4$ cup coconut butter
$1/2$ tsp. baking powder
Pinch salt

Mix all the ingredients for the crust in a large bowl. Lightly grease and flour a deep, oven-safe pie dish (9-inch dish recommended). Press the crust firmly into the pie dish and chill while you make the filling.

#### Filling

1 cup plain yogurt
2 cups blueberries, fresh or frozen
$2 1/2$ tbsp. sugar

2 tbsp. finely grated lemon zest

1 tbsp. lemon juice

1 tsp. vanilla

2 eggs

1 tbsp. flour

Place eggs in a large mixing bowl and beat until mixed thoroughly. Add the yogurt, sugar, lemon zest, juice, vanilla, and flour. Pour into the chilled pie crust and add blueberries last. Bake at 350°F for 50 minutes, or until pie filling turns to custard consistency. Let cool for 10 minutes and serve.

# SEVEN

# Peaks, Valleys,
## and Plateaus

FOR MANY YEARS, I thought that there would be a day when I would "arrive." I would arrive at the perfect body. I would arrive at the perfect weight. I would be fit, athletic, and healthy, and then once that happened, I could get off the treadmill and relax and enjoy my perfect body in my now-perfect life. Perhaps this has crossed your mind too? If I worked out rigorously enough and stuck to my diet, I could have it all. I thought this would be the key to my happiness.

Back then I was in an "all or nothing" mindset: "all" included exercising five days a week and eating mostly tuna and salad. When "all" became too difficult (my all was not sustainable), I threw in the towel and declared, "It's not working." This became an endless cycle. Can you relate?

I didn't view exercise as something I would always do. Like many of my attempts at getting healthy, my tactics had expiration dates: the thirty-day fitness challenge, the fourteen-day cleanse. These messages about short-term health investments are reiterated in women's health magazines and all around us. When you can "drop two dress sizes in twelve days" or experience "twenty-one days to a New You," why would you think a healthy lifestyle requires maintenance and long-term commitment? The realization that "getting healthy" is a lifelong process isn't an easy one, and it hit me pretty hard. I felt discouraged to think that I would always be climbing mountains.

After many years of being duped by every diet trick in the book, I realized fitness was not a temporary goal but an every-day necessity and that it required commitment. I found that commitment is actually enjoyable, but a healthy lifestyle isn't a mountain you climb once. Life as an athlete is full of peaks, valleys, and plateaus. You will never "arrive." Some days the workout really sucks and you feel like you can't go on. But other days you are a powerful ass-kicker. Those are the days that will keep you coming back for more. Everyone experiences difficult workouts they wish they'd never shown up for—but the problem arises when you judge yourself or allow yourself to get stuck. These valleys—times when you feel low—are not times to give up. They do not mean that you are a failure. Peaks, valleys, and plateaus are normal phases of the human experience, in fitness and in life, and you must not criticize yourself when you are in a valley. There are ways to pull yourself through every phase of the athlete's journey.

---

**Serena Williams, professional tennis player:**
"I really think a champion is defined not by their wins but by how they can recover when they fall."

---

In those down times you must remain positive. This means accepting where you are, being patient, and trusting in the process. Our bodies need our respect; as you increase physical stress on your body through exercise, it needs time to manage the load. One of my trainers once told me that difficult training sessions are "breaking your body down," and that is exactly right. When we put physical stress on the body, we break it down so that it can rebuild itself to be even stronger. This is how we gain muscle and improve fitness.

This process, sometimes called "break and build," is also known as "challenge and rest." Resting is just as important as exercising; our bodies need time to process, repair, and come back stronger for the next workout. When your body plateaus and you don't see any gains, it is saying, "I need a minute." If your best friend said, "I need to rest for a minute," you'd respect that. Would you yell "What's wrong with you?!" Why do we do that to ourselves? Respect your body's needs.

Let's look more closely at the different phases of performance.

## The Peak (AKA the Ass-Kicking Zone)

IN THE ASS-KICKING ZONE our bodies demonstrate their full potential, and we feel limitless: we can conquer the world, this workout, and the next. Peaks are exhilarating.

Peaks happen when everything lines up. We are ready—we have a good base of physical conditioning under our belts. We feel supported—those around us are encouraging us. And we are on an unstoppable path to our attainable goals.

Peaks are what we live for. You might be experiencing a peak if you are downward dogging it like no one's business in yoga class, walking hills at a newfound speed, and keeping up with the Zumba instructor's every step.

There's no mistaking when you're at the peak; it's in every fiber of your being.

Leanne Stewart is a plus-size athlete who knows what being in her peak zone feels like. Leanne says, "I always wanted to run.

I always thought my asthma and weight were roadblocks, and everyone else seemed much fitter than me. But an opportunity came up to join a 'Learn to Run' group that was at my pace."

Leanne started slow by running thirty seconds before walking for two minutes. She continued to run three times a week, increasing her run times as she went. "I was running! I was totally in the zone, high on endorphins and feeling like an accomplished athlete for the first time in my life. Each run session only propelled and motivated me to keep going. Before I knew it I was running seven minutes in a row."

As her endurance increased, Leanne's feelings of self-doubt dissipated, and she signed up for her first 5K. "The run day came and I was ready. I was excited. The run started and my pace steadied. I ran strong for the full 5K, and as I approached the finish line I saw my teammates and daughter standing waiting for me. I was so proud. I did it!"

Leanne experienced a peak while training for her first 5K race. She steadily progressed, felt motivated, and accomplished her goal. Peaks are not just reserved for those training for runs or races. Being in the zone, or at your athletic peak, can simply mean making it to your aerobics class each week and feeling energized and motivated enough to go back in two days and do it again. Being in the zone can mean meeting your neighbors on the corner every night and walking the neighborhood with energized conviction. Anything you do regularly and feel good about and want to continue doing can lead to athletic peaks.

You know you are in the zone when your inner monologue starts saying "Yes!" instead of "No," and when your self-talk has become positive: "You're on fire!" The peak is what we strive for and where we feel empowered to become consistent exercisers. However, we are also human beings who have good days and bad days. Life's psychological, emotional, and physical obstacles can sometimes send us into a valley.

## The Valley (AKA a Down Period)

YOU COME TO your workout feeling drained before you even begin; your motivation is just not there. In this period, which can feel frustrating, the negative chatter in your mind is at an all-time high and it's working to sabotage things even further. I might head out for a run because it's on my training schedule, but in a valley each step feels like I am moving through molasses. On this run, I might choose the path that leads to the shortcut rather than the one that pushes me to increase my distance.

You can enter a valley for a number of reasons—for example, from working out too much: overtraining can leave you feeling exhausted and cause you to fall out of your peak zone. Another example: you might be bored with your fitness routine. You may need to switch things up to keep motivated. Or you might be fighting a cold and not feeling well. Other reasons might include pressure from work, family commitments, or fear or anxiety that subconsciously tax your energy levels.

Every athlete will tell you they've been in a valley. Everyone feels off his or her game at some point. It's natural, and yet many of us use this as an opportunity to be hard on ourselves and sometimes quit.

I prefer to say "in the valley" to "falling off the wagon." For me, talking about falling off something indicates an all-or-nothing mentality: you are either on or you are off. A valley is a normal part of a journey: sometimes we climb mountains, and sometimes we walk in the valley. But after the valley, there will be another mountain and another high.

Jodene Blain is a plus-size runner. Time in the valley has been a part of her athletic path. Jodene says:

I am always amazed when I feel the valley low or hit the wall. My commitment can be unwavering for several months, all the time knowing that any changes in my schedule instantly make me feel uneasy. [The valley] can sneak up because of a weekend away, a common cold, or something as absurd as a goal accomplished, like when I complete a race. I lose my passion and enthusiasm despite feeling strong and successful. Over the years I have learned not to be too hard on myself. I now have the confidence to understand that muscle memory really exists, and as I begin again it only takes a few days to a week to find my stride and feel my strength return. I am a stronger person and better mom and partner when I exercise and commit to fitness goals, and I can't allow a temporary low to take that away from me.

## The Plateau (AKA a Steady State)

PERHAPS YOU ARE showing up for your workouts, eating healthy food, and getting a good night's sleep, but your physical fitness has not progressed. You wonder what you are doing wrong and why you aren't seeing better results. You feel frustrated and fragile.

A few things are happening during a plateau period. First, your body may no longer be challenged by your fitness routine. You might consider increasing the intensity of your workout or varying the type of activity you do. Second, your body might require a rest and is telling you to hit pause. Training programs often include scheduled recovery weeks, which allow time for your body to rest, rebuild, and prepare for another push. Plateaus are beneficial for the body—they are a natural response to the demand you place on your body with each workout.

How can you tell whether your body has adjusted to your workout and needs more intensity or whether your body is asking for rest? To figure that out, ask yourself how difficult your workout feels while you are doing it. If you feel that you can kick it up a notch and your body would meet you in that challenge, then you need to intensify your routine. If it feels as if your body might be maxed out no matter what activity you throw at it, then it is time to rest. Understanding your body's physical needs requires careful attention and should be taken seriously to avoid injury, exhaustion, or throwing in the towel.

I avoid plateaus in my own training and in the training I provide for my clients by developing programs that involve constant change. I watch clients closely and make sure their plateaus are not a result of their bodies adapting to their physical demand. I ensure they increase weights when needed and that they intensify their cardio by calling them out and encouraging them to step it up. Throughout my classes strength exercises are performed with a variety of equipment, and we work the major muscle groups in slightly different ways. I also mix up when we perform cardio and what we do to get our heart rates up so that each time my clients come to class they face a brand new challenge. I also keep a close watch on clients who need to go more slowly and tone down my push for them to perform so they can attend, but still exercise at a pace that works for them. When writing a program to meet an athletic goal, such as a half-marathon or triathlon, I ensure there are weeks when distance and exertion are dialed down a notch so that clients don't overexert their bodies. These are called plateau, taper, or recovery weeks.

If you have a trainer and are concerned that you have reached a plateau, ask him or her to help identify why you have stagnated. If your body needs rest, you may have to reduce the intensity of your workouts or introduce activities that require less exertion. If your body is looking for new challenges, mix it up!

If you work out alone (without a trainer), think of ways you can approach your training differently. In the pool, pick up the pace, add lengths, or swim at different paces (interval training) by alternating two fast laps with two slow laps. This gives the body a new challenge. If you are running or walking for fitness, move faster, add inclines, or increase your distance. And if you are not already doing this, introduce cross-training by adding a new sport or activity to your routine that allows you to work your muscles in a new way. This will enhance your performance in all of your workouts. For example, if your main activity is playing tennis, add weights at the gym to build muscle in your upper body. This will improve your return on the court. A runner might add cycling to target different leg muscles and to work the cardiovascular system in a different way.

Most athletes know the importance of listening to their body. You will come to know its language well. As you build a relationship with your body, you will learn the cues that indicate what is going well and what is not. It helps to keep a record of how each workout felt. Each day, record the activity you performed and answer the following questions by rating them from 1 to 10.

On a scale of 1–10:
- How did your workout feel today?
- Did you put forth your best effort?
- Did you have a good sleep?
- How is your nutrition?
- How is your hydration?
- How is your stress level?

FOR FEMALE ATHLETES, your menstrual cycle is also something to consider in athletic performance. Sessions can be more difficult during certain phases of your cycle. If you're feeling like you're in the valley or plateauing, also take note of where you are in your cycle. *Medical News Today* recently ran an article on menstruation and athletic performance, which agrees that our cycle can affect our ability to physically perform at our best: "These symptoms have a lot of potential to disrupt a sportswoman's performance. In addition to the cramping, women can experience other physical symptoms such as joint and muscle pain, headaches, weight gain and low energy levels."[1]

These common menstrual symptoms can all affect your athletic performance, and it is helpful to be aware of them.

You might feel happiest when you are making progress, but those times when you need to stay in the same place are just as important. They will be what move you further in the long run. It is counterproductive to beat yourself up during a plateau. Be kind to yourself and use positive language. Avoid language like, "I should be able to," "I wish I could," "I used to be able to," and "Why can't I?"

Also, try not to apologize for where you are at in your journey. I hear apologies a lot. Some of my clients feel they must apologize if they didn't complete an exercise or they needed to rest. I see them in all their sweaty glory rocking a workout, and then they trivialize their amazing work when they say, "Sorry." They assume that I am disappointed in them, that they have let me down or they have let themselves down.

No apology is needed; just being there is a huge accomplishment. This is hard stuff. There is nothing wrong with listening to your body and doing what is required in that moment. Do not apologize for your fitness. Ever.

My goal is to help clients do their best and understand and listen to their body; this is the model for a consistent long-term exerciser. I hope that by learning to listen to their bodies, my clients will learn to love them. I hope you do too. Our bodies are miracles. They do what we ask them to do. We train them, they work hard, and it isn't always easy. We must show compassion along the way.

If, while trying to work out, you find yourself saying, "But it's just not working," stop and ask yourself what "it" means, what "working" means. What is your definition of success? Be careful that you don't accidentally adopt the expectations that others place on you, including well-meaning family members and trainers. I worry that too often "working" means "losing weight." Not seeing the losses you expected can make you want to throw in the towel—I've done this too many times to count. And yet, we forget the amazing things we have accomplished, the gains we have made, when we give up. Maybe our vision of success needs to be rewritten. It can be helpful to write down what success means to you. To me, success means to establish goals, map out a plan, follow the plan, and accomplish my goals. Finish the race or learn to swim in the ocean—stepping on a scale is far from *my* version of success.

To weather the peaks, valleys, and plateaus of your athletic journey, you must base your success on more than just the numbers on the scale. You are in this for the long term, and exercise has many benefits that have nothing to do with what you weigh. Instead of throwing in the towel, throw out the scale. Take the energy you would spend obsessing about that number and refocus it on your healthy lifestyle and fitness goals.

Sometimes it's helpful to have barometers that you can use to measure your journey. Here are ten ways to measure your health and fitness achievements that do not involve the scale.

## 1. Psyche and Mood

EXERCISE MAKES YOU feel good. I notice almost immediately how much better people feel when they start exercising.
It was true for me too. Now I can tell when I need to work out.
I get what I call "stinking thinking": I become negative, impa-
tient, and stressed out. Exercise immediately gives me a better
outlook on life, and I instantly feel good about myself.

This good feeling is due to brain chemistry. As we increase
the demand on our bodies through exercise, the brain says,
"Hey, wait a minute, I feel some stress coming on." Our brains
think we are fighting off or fleeing the enemy and release a
protein called Brain-Derived Neurotropic Factor (BDNF). The
release of BDNF after exercise is coupled with the release of
endorphins, which make you feel euphoric. This is a great
reason to move our bodies! Increased endorphins can reduce
depression and anxiety and help manage stress—one of the
primary benefits of exercise in my life.

## 2. Sleep Patterns

EXERCISE HELPS MANY people sleep better. Physical activity
raises core body temperature, and as it slowly declines it sig-
nals to the body that it is time to prepare for rest. For someone
like me, who can sleep at a rock concert, this isn't a huge benefit, but for those who have difficulty falling asleep or staying
asleep, exercise can be a lifesaver.

If you are someone who has difficulty sleeping, exercise
right before bed might not be the best idea. It's hard to sleep
when you're high on endorphins! Give yourself some time to
wind down before bed. Take a bath, read a book, or just sit qui-
etly for at least thirty minutes before lights out.

An athletic lifestyle must include adequate rest. I often get
asked, "How do you do it all?" My answer is that I go to bed

most nights at nine o'clock. My days start really early and they are action-packed, but by nine, I am ready for deep rest. I look forward to going to bed, and I sleep deeply every night. Exercise also reduces stress, which affects how well we sleep.

## 3. Bone Density

FOR WOMEN, ESPECIALLY, the impact of exercise on bones is a big deal. Bones are living organs, and we experience new bone growth and lose old bone just like we shed skin cells. When we are young, we develop new bone growth more rapidly. Around age thirty, our bones hit their highest bone mass, also known as peak bone mass. Between thirty and peri-menopause (which often begins in our forties) bone mass decreases slightly, but after peri-menopause and beyond bone mass can decline quickly, which may lead to osteoporosis. Healthfully stressing our bones through exercise promotes bone density, which protects us from fracture as well as osteoporosis. It is especially important to exercise as our bone density decreases, but exercise is also an important preventative measure we can start in early adulthood.

## 4. Self-Esteem and Confidence

WHEN I EXERCISE regularly, I have increased self-esteem, I am more confident, and I am better able to reach my highest potential in all areas of my life. Because of this I try to reinforce the importance of physical activity in my son's life. The earlier we start being active, the more natural it is to live an active lifestyle. At nine years old, my son is a very confident boy. He does not excel at all the sports he is involved in, but just participating is an important building block for his self-esteem.

According to a recent study in the *Journal of Health Psychology*, people with a low sense of self-confidence gained greater confidence not from how hard they exercised, how fast they ran, or how much they benched, but rather from whether they exercised at all.[2] It was the act of exercising that increased self-confidence, not how well they performed in the process.

The researchers reviewed fifty-seven case studies that looked into how regular exercise affected moods and emotional health. While they found that regular exercise did affect self-perceptions and self-confidence levels, there was no measurable difference between those who exercised moderately or intensely or between those who exercised for short periods or long periods. It did not matter what kind of activity people did during their exercise sessions either.

This study is not a one-off. Many studies both adults and children demonstrate that being physically active elevates self-esteem and self-confidence without the presence of weight loss. As your fitness improves, you realize how much you are capable of, thus increasing your feelings of self-worth.

## 5. Energy and Productivity

AS SOON AS my son was born and I was healed from my C-section, I began running again. People around me said, "Are you crazy? Aren't you too tired to run?" I *was* exhausted. Being a new mom didn't come naturally to me at all. But I needed to run; running helped me manage it all. After a run, I would come home energized and better equipped to be a good mom. I felt like myself when I ran. Running gave me the energy to do all the daily tasks involved in caring for a newborn.

When we exercise, we increase blood flow, and this increased blood flow helps deliver more oxygen throughout our bodies. The increased oxygen in turn creates more energy. As a result, after a workout, you are likely to feel much more energetic. Exercise also releases endorphins, which, as mentioned before, make us feel good. Sign me up!

I hear the "I'm too tired" excuse a lot. If you find yourself using this excuse, I encourage you to see if exercise will in fact give you more energy and motivate you to do more. I suspect you will see that I am right; the women who leave my classes are energetic, full of conversation and laughter. They may come to me feeling the effects of their day, but they leave lighter and happier, with the energy to finish the day strong.

## 6. Cardiovascular Health

REGULAR EXERCISE BUILDS good cardiovascular health. Good cardiovascular health doesn't just mean you can run farther or swim more laps. It means you can effortlessly climb a flight of stairs or run after your kids. Continued exercise strengthens the efficiency of your heart, making it possible for you to accomplish regular daily activities with less physical effort. The heart is a muscle, and as with other muscles, the more you exercise, the more strain you put on it, thus making it stronger.

The measure of improved cardio is in the recovery. When your cardiovascular system is strong, your recovery time will be seconds. When it isn't as strong, you need longer to recover.

## 7. Physical Strength and Endurance

I ONCE HAD a client whose goal was to get out of a chair. She was about to become a grandmother, and she was worried that she wouldn't be able to get out of a chair while holding her new grandchild. You may have heard the term "functional fitness"; it refers to your ability to complete the physical activities necessary for functioning in everyday life. Improving your functional fitness improves your quality of life, especially as you get older. For this particular client, not being able to get out of a chair meant she couldn't hold her grandson as she liked. Fitness isn't just about running races; we also need it to live life to its fullest. Working out increases your functionality, which allows you to participate in life more fully and independently no matter how old you are.

## 8. Active, Enriched Relationships

LIVING AN ACTIVE life attracts other active people. Often these people are goal-oriented positive thinkers and doers, and once you meet them there is much that you can share with one another. Before my own life was transformed I wanted to go on hikes, join fitness groups, and be adventurous, but I didn't have anyone to do it with. Now I can share amazing moments on top of mountains or crossing the finish line after cycling for two days with friends who share my interests. It's amazing to have friends who will go the miles with me. Sharing these adventures with them has deepened our relationships because we've trudged through challenging times together and come out on the other side, smiling.

Active living also enhances the relationships you can have with your family by making you a good role model. I want to model for my son that it is normal to get up early in the morning and exercise. Being fit has made possible incredible experiences that I want to share with my family.

## 9. Cognitive Health

EXERCISE HAS BEEN shown to improve brain health, especially for those between the ages of twenty-five and forty-five. Exercise boosts the chemicals in the brain that support and prevent degeneration of the hippocampus, the part of the brain responsible for memory and learning. In a paper published in 2014 in the online publication *Neurology*,[3] researchers at the University of Minnesota reported that young adults who run or participate in aerobic activities preserve their thinking and memory skills longer. Many more studies conclude that exercise increases brain function, not only as we get older, but also in the present day. Although you may not be thinking of your golden years just yet, building a solid foundation of physical fitness has been proven to improve your quality of life now and in the future.

## 10. Inspiration

I'VE DISCUSSED HOW women of size are rarely seen in athletic roles in media and advertising. As a result, many women believe they are alone in their desire to be an athlete. We need to show up, defy the stereotype of the unfit plus-size woman, and sweat it out to provide inspiration to others just joining the Big Fit Girl movement. You can be a part of this change by calling for representation in media and advertising. When you inspire someone simply with the choices you make and how you move through the world, you can change someone's life. You become an ambassador for what is possible.

THESE BENEFITS OF fitness are the tip of the iceberg. We may live in a culture that emphasizes fitness for the sake of thinness (and conforming to a set standard), but the reasons to be fit that we have examined here are much more powerful and positive than fitting into a smaller-sized dress. Exercise allows you to say yes; you will have the confidence and strength to show up and live your athletic dreams in the body you have now. It really can be a limitless life.

Remember, you are not alone. Putting yourself out there requires vulnerability, but the more of us who do it, who show up with varying abilities and in various sizes to celebrate the peaks, valleys, and plateaus, the more we convince the world and ourselves of our potential.

# Big Fit Girl
## Top-Twenty Playlist

Music is a great motivator, especially on those days when you just don't feel like getting out there and sweating. Research consistently shows that listening to music distracts athletes from their "bodily awareness" and helps them overcome discomfort. Studies also show that music at a fast tempo excites the brain and spurs the body to move. And it keeps you in the zone.

I like to listen to hard-driving, heart-pumping music. When one of my favorite songs comes on, I unconsciously work harder and go faster. I also feel more energized and empowered.

Here are my top twenty "go-to" songs for my fitness classes and personal workouts. If my list doesn't suit your taste, make your own with your favorite songs or search on the internet for the top workout songs.

All of the songs in my playlist can be found on iTunes.

1. **"Can't Stop the Feeling"**
   Justin Timberlake
2. **"Lose Yourself"**
   Eminem
3. **"Love Me Again"**
   John Newman
4. **"The Edge of Glory"**
   Lady Gaga
5. **"Wild Ones"**
   Flo Rida ft. Sia
6. **"Part of Me"**
   Katy Perry
7. **"Wake Me Up"**
   Avicii

8. **"Locked Out of Heaven"**
   Bruno Mars
9. **"Pump It"**
   The Black Eyed Peas
10. **"Thunderstruck"**
    AC/DC
11. **"Raise Your Glass"**
    Pink
12. **"Safe and Sound"**
    Capital Cities
13. **"Titanium"**
    David Guetta ft. Sia
14. **"Praise You"**
    Fatboy Slim
15. **"Suicide Blonde"**
    INXS
16. **"I Love It"**
    Icona Pop ft. Charli XCX
17. **"Sex on Fire"**
    Kings of Leon
18. **"Hey Ya!"**
    OutKast
19. **"Dancing with Myself"**
    Billy Idol
20. **"Confident"**
    Demi Lovato

Enjoy this playlist and keep rocking each workout!

# EIGHT

# Paying It Forward

WHAT WOULD IT look like to live in a world where, no matter your size or weight, you were encouraged to be fit and to work out at gyms and participate in sports and other physical activities? Imagine being accepted in athletics and treated with respect. What if you were welcomed with a smile and you had the confidence to sweat in any environment? Finding people who will champion your dreams is priceless, and their support is one of the most important things you need to achieve your highest athletic potential. But without this imaginary world where exercise is encouraged at any size, having a team in place to support you is crucial.

I have talked about my first run leader, Chris, and the profound impact she has had on my life. Seeing just one representation of a body that looked like mine in athletics became the catalyst for changing everything in my life: my outlook, my confidence, my friends, my health, and my career. I am so grateful to Chris for her courage to be seen as a plus-size athlete. While writing this book, I tracked her down through the store where she used to work and wrote her a long letter describing the impact she has had on my life. I told her about the things I am doing to help other women find their inner athlete.

She hadn't realized how she had influenced me and was blown away. She didn't know that in leading the group she was in fact paying it forward and making space for women like me to grow into leaders. When we all show up, and encourage others to show up, we break the norm, and that is valuable to those who wait on the sidelines.

## How Paying It Forward Is Beneficial to New Athletes

IT IS IMPORTANT for plus-size women to see themselves represented in athletics. When I started running, I was bigger than everyone in my group, and it caused me a great deal of anxiety. Seeing Chris, also a plus-size woman, encouraged me because I saw it was possible for me to be a runner. I realized that I wasn't limited by my size.

When you show up as an athlete, other plus-size women will benefit from your experience. I've had many trainers, leaders, and coaches, but Chris was different. She had already experienced what it felt like, both physically and emotionally, to break into the running world in a larger body. Other coaches I'd had were great, but they didn't understand the challenges that plus-size women face or what we are capable of.

There is most definitely strength in numbers. When we see more plus-size athletes and leaders in the fitness community, it starts to change what athleticism looks like. I remember getting certified as a fitness professional in a room full of muscular, ripped-looking athletes, and it was absolutely terrifying. But I've come to recognize that going through with my certification was an act of activism and part of the bigger picture. You can be a part of that big picture too.

Consider this part of your journey: when you find your inner athlete, pay it forward to those who are afraid to join in. You could be the reason someone's life dramatically changes. I can't express enough how enriching that experience will be for you.

## How Paying It Forward Is Beneficial for You

PAYING IT FORWARD also enriches *your* life. Sharing my athletic experiences with others has been one of the most rewarding experiences of my life. Giving back what was given to me fills my soul like nothing else. As I watch people achieve their goals—goals they thought were impossible to achieve—I am altered too.

Coaching others to help them achieve their goals has been a great learning experience for me. It has taught me that with the right training plan and with encouragement and support, all bodies are capable of anything. It has taught me patience, compassion, and how to support others.

Paying it forward is a gift and something I consider a privilege. When I started volunteering as a run leader, I had no intention of leaving my successful career to become fitness certified and coach women for a living. But the work was rewarding, and as time went on I realized I couldn't imagine doing anything else. Making this decision changed my life. You don't have to change careers to become an athletic leader and experience the change that paying it forward can bring. Big or small acts of paying it forward will change your outlook on life.

Your example could help others feel comfortable when joining a fitness program; those who come after you need to see women like themselves being active and achieving their fitness goals. When you are there to extend a hand and to show women the ropes of fitness and offer comfort, knowledge, or your own experiences, you become a mentor. You can guide people who aspire to walk in your shoes because you understand their challenges.

My friend Debbie is an Ironman triathlete. She has taken me for coffee to talk about the ins and outs of triathlons. They have a set of fairly strict rules that Debbie has taken the time to make sure I know. She has pointed me in the direction of pertinent websites, books, and videos that support triathlon racing and is there for me when I have questions. Debbie is a mentor to me, though we don't have an official agreement. She is just one athlete helping another. Most people who are paying it forward have overcome adversity themselves and are passionate about giving back.

This is how professional dancer and advocate Amanda Trusty found her way to giving back through dance.

As a young girl, Amanda was found dancing in malls, grocery aisles, and living rooms long before her mom finally bought her a blue leotard and stuck her in Miss Tina's dance class in West Lawn, Pennsylvania. She was only three years old, and her parents couldn't stop her from singing, shuffling, or wiggling. Since that day she hasn't stopped dancing.

Amanda started dancing competitively at age twelve and started doing community theater at age fifteen. These activities eventually led her to the stage in New York. She's now been in show business for as long as she can remember.

Until she started dancing competitively, Trusty was unaware that her body was different—larger and outside the norm of what most dancers looked like. This was when she met the older girls, the teens. Or as she describes them,

> The most beautiful girls on the planet who I looked up to so much and wanted to emulate so badly. It was in the back room where we kept all our shoes and where we ate meals between

classes that I learned about cellulite, birth control, and the pooch pouch. Everyone hated their lower belly, the pooch pouch. I came to learn that I had a really bad one. I didn't have a flat stomach, so my teacher would announce that we had to avoid two-piece costumes because of me. Not only were we screamed at and belittled in dance class, but my teacher made it very clear that my body was something to be ashamed of.

Although dancing itself brought Amanda tremendous joy, the criticisms behind the curtain have had devastating consequences. She experienced low self-esteem, disordered eating, and a constant feeling of not being good enough.

Amanda took her advocacy public when she created a dance video that went viral on YouTube. In her burlesque piece, she dances to Katy Perry's "Roar" and strips down to her underwear while also stripping away pieces of tape carrying negative comments about her body. These comments were those directed at her when she was a young dancer. Her video received more than a million views, and Amanda received support and thanks from around the world.

Amanda continues to pay it forward by giving body-positive dance classes to young girls and by writing for major publications, where she shares her struggles with body image. Her mission is to change dance culture and the stringent expectations of body conformity found there, and to allow women and girls to connect with their bodies in a joyful way through artistic expression.

---

**Muhammad Ali, professional boxer and historical icon:**
"Service to others is the rent you pay for your room here on earth."

---

When people experience their own personal revolution, it is natural to want to share that experience so that others can benefit from it too. We see the profound effects of paying it forward in examples such as twelve-step programs, where an experienced member sponsors a newcomer by taking on the role of guide and helping them get through their early days of recovery. This mentorship has a crucial impact on each person's ability to stick with the program.

There are many organizations, both non-profit and profit, that have a give-back component that counts toward the success of their business. Businesses that pay it forward with a social mission or impact are very much on-trend, and this policy often improves their bottom line. People like to see others championing those in need; it just feels good.

The greatest way you can give back is by showing up and being the change yourself. You can also start by being welcoming to others who join your gym or participate in a class you are taking. I see this with my clients; the apprehension disappears from the faces of newcomers when they receive encouragement and support from other members of the group. When we create an environment of inclusion, people let down their guard and participate.

Denise is a plus-size woman who found her inner athlete. Her athletic journey started with an office walking challenge where participants monitored the number of steps they took in a day. She went from taking three thousand steps a day to over ten thousand. Small steps literally led to big change. Because of her accomplishments, Denise was featured in the company's national newsletter, where she was able to pay it forward by telling her story. She opened up about her life and was willing to be seen and heard, offering an example to help others on their own journey. The day after the newsletter was released, Denise received forty-five emails from across the country sent by inspired co-workers within her company. Denise made a dramatic physical and mental transformation, one step at a time, and it increased her confidence. Soon she started running and joined our size-friendly boot camp. She says, "I don't really know if I had a dormant athlete lying in wait deep inside for fifty-five years. I kind of have the feeling I may have been someone who needed to create my inner athlete piece by piece. I had to learn to trust that I could try something new and have faith that eventually I would learn to enjoy doing it if I gave it time and consistent effort."

In the past, Denise hadn't committed to any fitness regime long enough to get past her initial resistance. She needed an instructor and a tribe who could push her past this crucial point and help her through her negative feelings. When she came to me, I knew that Denise wanted to become an athlete and that she was looking for someone to show her the path. "I needed mentorship," Denise says. "I needed to say, 'I am an athlete' over and over until I heard it enough times I began to understand that it applied to me. I started to see that when I changed my thinking about myself, people around me started seeing and treating me differently too." In the end, she was able to change her way of thinking and her attitude toward fitness.

Denise offers a warm smile to newcomers to our group. She always extends a hand to others. She says, "My advice to anyone starting is to give it some time. Commit to the length of time you'll need to actually make progress. Go long enough so you experience people coming to class who are newer than you are. When you are no longer the visitor or feeling like the invader, then you can turn around and help make the newly-joined feel welcome and part of the tribe. You understand how they feel. You understand because you have traveled the road and put in your time and are now an athlete."

If you find yourself in a position of leadership, as others come to you for advice, take the opportunity to make an impact on another person's journey. My experiences have shown me that giving back is extremely enriching for both parties. Here are some ways to pay it forward and to experience the joy of helping others find their greatest potential.

## Paying It Forward in Your Community

- Readily share your experiences with others. Don't hide your background and knowledge. You have valuable information and inspiration to offer those around you. When people ask, tell them what you are doing and how you are staying motivated. Invite them to join you. Often people will engage in fitness when they can do it with a supportive friend. Be that friend.
- Start a walking, running, or cycling group. When people feel they have a safe place to go, they will show up. Walking in your neighborhood offers an opportunity for everyone to come out. It's free and accessible to many people. It will be inspiring to both you and the new walker. Walking or running groups are social and create opportunities to develop active friendships.
- Write about your experiences. Whether you do this on social media or create your own personal blog, you can offer information on how to get started and share your own story for inspiration. Plus-size women are still grossly underrepresented, so showing what can be done in bodies of all shapes and sizes can make a profound impression on many people.
- Offer your wholehearted opinion. If people ask what's missing in the fitness industry for women of size, don't be afraid to tell them. Sharing your thoughts creates change. I am often asked to provide an expert opinion on fitness for plus-size women for articles, radio, and television segments. I don't hold back on anything! Speaking the truth is the only way we can create change.

- Show up. Seeing more plus-size women working out is the most important factor in changing people's perceptions of what an athlete might look like. Until we have better representation of bodies in advertising and the media, we have to do this for one another.

- Welcome others. Greet newcomers to your fitness class or program with a smile and share your experiences with them. You might be surprised at how far a warm smile and authentic encouragement can go. When people hear that you too were afraid in the beginning but that you overcame the fear, they will feel encouraged to do the same. Knowing that they will see a friendly face when they arrive at class takes away most of their anxiety and can make the difference in whether someone returns or not.

- Obtain your fitness certification to lead others. Some of you may feel so passionate about helping others that you will decide to get your fitness certification. I remember sharing my fears about being a plus-size trainer with my neighbor, and she said that was exactly the reason she would want to work with me. People want to be supported by people they can relate to. When you and your client have shared a similar experience, the bond of trust runs deep. Simply by showing up in my larger body, I can put a client at ease. I am familiar with the obstacles they are facing, because I have lived through them myself. The personal experience I share with my clients allows me to be a better support person for them.

- Volunteer at fitness events. You can enjoy the fun and inspiration of a sporting event while also helping other athletes. One of my most inspirational memories is cheering the athletes on at Ironman Canada. I was so inspired that some moments I was moved to tears. After fifteen hours on the course, the athletes were so grateful to hear our words of encouragement as they ran by. Giving back and supporting others is without doubt a win/win. Seeing those men and women compete made me want to push harder and go further in my own triathlon journey.

- Deliver a talk about your experience. People—especially people of size—are hungry for inspiration and new information about health and wellness because information that pertains specifically to bigger bodies in fitness is lacking. Libraries and coffee shops are a great place to start a grassroots speakers' night that could include personal fitness stories—which are always inspiring—followed by an evening walk. I have hosted several events at plus-size retailers where I shared my journey as a plus-size athlete. I promoted the events on social media and made posters to draw people in. People came to hear me speak, and afterwards we headed outside for a twenty-minute walk. It always made for a great evening because people can get inspired by the talk and then get some exercise, which can ignite motivation to get started. It is up to us to take every opportunity to be seen and heard to inspire others. Make yourself known, and the people will follow.

SOME OF MY biggest inspirations came from people giving back through groundbreaking books from authors who share their experiences. Here are some of the best body-positive books on the market:

## My Top Seven Books from Authors Giving Back

1. *Things No One Will Tell Fat Girls: A Handbook for Unapologetic Living*
   Jes Baker
   Seal Press, 2015

2. *Triathlon for the Every Woman: You Can Be a Triathlete. Yes. You.*
   Meredith Atwood
   Tricycle Books, 2012
3. *Gorge: My Journey Up Kilimanjaro at 300 Pounds*
   Kara Richardson Whitely
   Seal Press, 2015
4. *Slow Fat Triathlete: Live Your Athletic Dreams in the Body You Have Now*
   Jayne Williams
   Da Capo Press, 2004
5. *Fat Girl Walking: Sex, Food, Love, and Being Comfortable in Your Skin . . . Every Inch of It*
   Brittany Gibbons
   Dey Street Books, 2015
6. *Embrace: My Story from Body Loather to Body Lover*
   Taryn Brumfitt
   New Holland Publishers, 2015
7. *The Gifts of Imperfection: Let Go of Who You Think You're Supposed to Be and Embrace Who You Are*
   Brené Brown
   Hazelden, 2010

AS A NEW athlete I read Jayne Williams's book, and it fired me up to keep going. The women who wrote the books listed are leaders giving back to women looking for inspiration.

You can inspire, too, and feel the rewards. One way to do that is join a community that offers support to plus-size athletes.

## Giving Back Online

FACEBOOK OFFERS THE opportunity to join or create a closed or private group so that you can network with other women on a similar journey. Here are five of my favorite groups. You can join one or start your own.

1. Fit Fatties

   Fit Fatties is a closed forum on Facebook created by Ragen Chastain and Jeanette DePatie. This group is a Health at Every Size group and is strictly weight neutral, meaning absolutely no weight-loss talk, no diet talk, and no negative body talk for any reason. If you are interested in joining this forum, you can send a request to the administrators of the page.

2. Body Positive Athletes

   Body Positive Athletes is a closed Facebook group and a blog founded by Leah Gilbert. Leah and hundreds of other athletes from around the globe share their athletic experiences and tips with others in the group. It's a great place to ask questions and get some solid answers from those who approach fitness with a body-positive perspective.

3. Athena Triathletes

   This is a private Facebook group for triathletes who compete as or empathize with triathletes in the Athena class (165+ pounds). A request to join is required; this is a forum where many women triathletes share their experiences and tips and support one another.

4. Born to Reign Athletics

   Born to Reign is a Facebook page by triathlete Krista Henderson. The entire page is geared toward plus-size athleticism in many forms and includes great resources for and information about finding your inner athlete.

5. Body Positive Yoga

   Body Positive Yoga, founded by Amber Karnes, is a Facebook page and business where students of all shapes and sizes will find tips, tricks, and modifications to make yoga asana work for their unique body. Amber pays it forward through her classes, online community, and yoga training program.

IF YOU PLAN to start an online community, here are some things to consider before getting started:

- What is the purpose of the forum or community?
- Who is it intended for?
- What are the ground rules for appropriate language and comments?
- Do you have a code of conduct? If so, add it to your description.
- Do you have a strategy for how to create a safe place? You should monitor your community regularly.
- Will you be involved in the community? You should engage regularly with its members.

## Giving Back in Person

AT THE BACK of this book you will find a 5K training program for both walkers and runners. You don't have to be an official run leader to organize a group in your community.

Several years ago I started a 10K clinic in Vancouver's Downtown Eastside. This area of our city is one of Canada's most underprivileged neighborhoods, and many of the runners who signed up were HIV positive, mentally ill, or struggling with drug addiction. Fifty-two people signed up in a neighborhood where running programs simply didn't exist.

The training program lasted for thirteen weeks, and over time some of the participants helped us lead the group. Those who took on leadership roles seemed to be the most committed to crossing the finish line thirteen weeks later. Their participation as leaders also kept their peers interested and held them accountable to keep coming, and by the end of the program we had thirty-seven people cross the finish line of a 10K race! The program got the community involved and working toward positive goals together. The program has been passed on and has been running successfully since 2010, providing our most vulnerable citizens with the opportunity to experience endorphins, sweat, and victory. This was one of the most enriching experiences of my career. Paying it forward rewards everyone.

There is great dignity and purpose in showing up for others, and you don't have to be a certified coach or other expert to do it. You just have to have the passion and the heart.

Here are some things to consider when starting an offline group, whether it's a walking, running, swimming, or biking group or a speaker series:

- Reliability
  As the leader of the group, your reliability is key because others are looking to you for accountability. In my role as a fitness leader, there have been times when I didn't want to teach an outdoor winter class, but it's my job, and regardless of what I want, I need to show up for the people I've committed to. This applies to my volunteer work, too. If you can't imagine yourself following through with the group, it's best not to start.
- Good Communication and Organization
  Most groups will need good group communication and organization. You will need to provide some direction. As the leader you are often responsible for setting up meeting

times, communicating what the workout is (the run, walk, swim, hike, whatever your group does). As the leader you will want to make sure your community is clear on what is happening. I've been out on group runs where everyone was confused on which way to go, and it was extremely frustrating.

- Sharing

Sharing your own experience is integral to paying it forward because it establishes a sense of trust and understanding and it shows others that you know how they feel. When people share common ground it creates connection. Be ready to tell others about the obstacles you faced and what worked and didn't work as you met each goal. Your stories will inspire others, help them relate, and allow them to see their own possibilities through your journey.

- Recruiting

To recruit people for your group, you will need to spread the word. Tell your friends, family, neighbors, and co-workers. Before I became certified I sent out an inter-office email and asked my colleagues if they wanted to join my 5K run program. I was surprised that many of them did. We trained together for weeks and then met our end goal of a 5K race. It brought us closer together as co-workers and many of them are still running.

- Delegating

You want your group to remain a passion project and something that brings you satisfaction. If it becomes too much, you will likely start to resent it. Delegate tasks to other group members or find a co-leader now or along the way. Taking on a leadership role enables you to take part in changing people's perceptions of plus-size women in fitness. Those who have come before us to pay it forward have set us a great example. Now we must grab the reins and lead.

LEAH GILBERT IS a plus-size endurance athlete who sees paying it forward as a big part of her success and takes great pride in her career as a coach.

> I can honestly say that one of the core motivations for what I do is to see people flourish as a result of realizing their own athletic potential. It's a privilege to see that exact moment when a person you have been working with becomes fearless and just goes for it. I coached one of my clients into her first triathlon, and she hasn't looked back; in fact we will probably now train and race together this season. I don't aim to build a relationship of dependence with my clients; I aim to help set the foundations for them to build their own experiences upon. It's like nurturing a bird with the aim of releasing it back into the wild—you care for it, make it strong, and help it realize it can fly again. And that moment that it flies off into the great unknown with strength and confidence—well, that's your moment right there.

Helping a fellow human being is an important mission, and it can be infectious. I invite you on this beautiful journey of changing the world one smile and pat on the back at a time.

I have transformed my life from one of wallowing in self-pity and being stuck in a pattern of unhealthy living, to existing as a terrified exerciser who thought she was too big, too slow, and just plain out of place, to being someone who has smashed every stereotype there is. I found my inner athlete and have built a movement for others to join, or find their own. I find great power in paying it forward.

My journey continues each and every day as I continue to grow. Yours will too.

This is that moment when our limitless potential is unleashed. As you head into your life as a Big Fit Girl, keep the following principles of this book in mind:

- You can unleash your inner athlete no matter what your size.
- You are the CEO of your body and no one but you gets to decide what is best for it. Only the best of the best are allowed on your team—make sure that happens.
- The right gear is out there for your endeavors. Just find it using the information in this book and then go rock it out!
- Set goals. You are worth achieving your aspirations—every single one of them. Remember to be SMART. Mapping out your goals will bring you closer to your limitless life.
- Food doesn't have to be the enemy. Use it to give you energy on your path to limitless living. Forget about restricting foods; just give your body what it needs, in healthy abundance, and enjoy all foods.
- Your road as an athlete will have peaks, valleys, and plateaus; they are all part of the journey. You will weather the storms.
- When you've got it, you must give it back. Paying it forward comes with great rewards to both you and the new athlete. This is how Big Fit Girls will change the face of athleticism for all. This is how we become limitless.

You are now part of a global movement of Big Fit Girls creating change, one workout at a time. Be free, reign like an athlete, and live limitlessly. It's your time.

# ACKNOWLEDGMENTS

WOULD LIKE TO acknowledge all the believers, supporters, and champions behind *Big Fit Girl*. Without you, this book would not have been possible.

A very special acknowledgment goes to Nancy Flight of Greystone Books for seeing the need for *Big Fit Girl*. When many people said no, you said yes, and I am eternally grateful to you for understanding the importance of this book's message. Your insight will forever change the fitness bookshelves for big girls, far and wide.

My gratitude and acknowledgment goes out to the entire team at Greystone Books: you set the bar high and I love you for it.

A huge shout-out to my agent, Jesse Finkelstein—your endless support means the world to me; and to my quasi advisors Jes Baker, Karen Bannister, and Amanda Edwards—thank you for your words of wisdom and professional input.

Sending big love and gratitude to all the brave women who shared their stories in *Big Fit Girl*. Your experiences of struggle and triumph as big girls navigating the fitness industry will help many women through their own athletic journeys, and that is a big gift to the world. Thank you.

To the professional experts who took time out of their busy schedules to back my book and share their valuable insights, thank you!

My endless gratitude goes out to the body-positive advocates and activists who have championed my message (and their own) and who have shown me it's okay to be brave and stand up for what I believe in, unapologetically.

To my good friend Tarryn Rudolph and all my Body Exchange ladies, your support has been immeasurable; you are some of the finest Big Fit Girls I know.

Thank you to my mom and dad and my Liverpool roots for giving me a strong voice to stand up for what I believe in.

Last but not least, a huge thank-you to my husband, Gord, and my son, Eli, for understanding that Mom needs to follow her dreams, and while that takes a lot of time away from you, your understanding and support helps move our society closer to becoming a more accepting place for every "body." I love you both beyond words.

# 5K for Every Body: Learn to Run or Walk Program

LEARNING TO RUN a 5K distance is where it all started for me, and it changed my life. Maybe it can change yours too?

I have created a 5K program that has been used for hundreds of plus-size 5K participants. Some 5K programs start off too aggressively with participants running for a full minute. My program is based on the assumption that exercise might be a brand-new undertaking and that walking or running plus-size may require extra safety precautions.

Whether you are interested in walking or running, this is a great place to start. What I love about training people to complete a 5K distance is the incredible progress that is so apparent as you move along. This program is easy to follow, it's free, and you can do the workouts when it's convenient for you.

TAKE THE TIME to review the program, and consider creating a tribe to join you. Accountability and support will be key.

Following is some of the terminology used throughout this program. Familiarize yourself with the program and then set a date to start training:

- *Warm-up:*
  The "warm-up" in this program is simply a five-minute moderately-paced walk. Whether you plan to use this program as a walking plan or a running plan, every participant should start with a gradual warm-up.
- *Cool-down:*
  Like the warmup, the "cool-down" is a five-minute moderately paced walk. This allows for your heart rate and breathing to gradually return to their resting rate and gives your muscles time to return to their optimal length and tension.
- *Slow interval:*
  Throughout this program the term "slow interval" is used to refer to the recovery interval. During this interval you walk slowly or moderately to recover from the fast interval.
- *Fast interval:*
  Through out this program you will also see the term "fast interval." This term means something different for those who wish to run 5K and for those who wish to walk it. If you are learning to walk a 5K, the fast interval is a faster-paced walk than the slow interval. This increases your stamina and endurance by pushing the cardiovascular system to build strength to finish the race. If you plan to use this program to learn how to run a 5K distance, then the fast interval means you will run during this time.
- *Low and slow:*
  "Low and slow" means to run with little impact at a slow pace, almost like a shuffle. When you shuffle the run, it leaves little room for impact and protects your joints. Running slowly preserves energy, and when you are starting out, this is really important. The goal is to get you through each interval successfully. Start off running low and slow and then increase your pace when you feel you can.

- *Total time:*
  "Total time" refers to the total time out per training session. This time includes the five-minute warm-up and the five-minute cool-down. As time goes on in the program, you will notice that your "time out" increases and your fast intervals get longer too. This allows for a gradual build.
- *Long run or walk:*
  Within most running programs there is what's called a "long run." Throughout the week you will have two or three shorter runs, called tempo runs, and one long run. The long run builds endurance so that you have the gas to complete the distance. The long run is typically the run that is done with your clinic group, although some groups do all their runs together.
- *Tempo run or walk:*
  A "tempo run" is usually a shorter run that is performed at a faster pace. When I started running, I only had one pace. Don't worry too much about these paces in the beginning. I just want you out there comfortably completing each session.
- *Homework:*
  "Homework" refers to the runs that will be done on your own, usually mid-week tempo runs. This structure is usually what is found in a true running clinic but I strongly urge you to find a group that you can be accountable to for all of your runs (or walks).
- *Conditioning phase:*
  "Conditioning phase" usually refers to the beginning of a program or a pre-program phase. Some people who haven't run before might find their bodies rebel against this new activity. You may become very sore or fatigued if you don't follow an appropriate program. The conditioning phase allows you to ease in very gradually to "condition" your body for the program ahead. It's a very important phase.

- *Recovery week:*
  The "recovery week" in the program is one where you will see no increases in your run or walk schedule. This gives your body a chance to recover and catch up and reaffirm the demands placed on it. The following week you will begin increasing again, so use this recovery week to go slow and easy to prepare for what is next.
- *Race day:*
  I always recommend that people seek out an event or race that hosts a 5K fun run or walk before they start the program. Once you have signed up it seals the deal on your commitment. A "race day" event is a fantastic way to celebrate your amazing accomplishment.

AS YOU REVIEW my program, you may wonder why certain sessions are longer than others, why we taper in the end, and why we recover mid-program. There is a method to the madness, and this program is designed from my experiences out in the field. You may be tempted to jump ahead because running for thirty seconds feels too easy. I urge you to follow the program because each session is there for a reason: to slowly develop your ability to run 5K without injury.

Here are some basic tips for reaching the finish line:

- Keep your pace slow for low impact and try to use as little energy as possible.
- Pump your arms when you hit any inclines, whether walking or running; this helps build momentum in your legs.
- Follow the program, even if it seems boring in the beginning.
- Don't get discouraged by looking ahead at the plan. Every person I've trained is in total disbelief that they can finish the plan, but they do!
- Hydrate before, during, and after your run/walk sessions.
- Fuel with healthy food.

- Try to push negative thinking out of your mind. When things get tough, come up with a mantra that cheers you on, like: "I am a strong and capable athlete!"
- Stretch after each session. You can find a stretching routine in Appendix B (p. 191).
- Make sure that you have good, properly fitted shoes.
- Have fun! Find a group of friends and unleash your inner athlete.

HERE WE GO:

## 5K FOR EVERY BODY

| Week | Fast Interval<br>Run or Fast Walk | Slow Interval<br>Moderate Walk | Quantity<br>How many times this combo is repeated | Check List<br>Stay on track and check when complete | Total Time<br>Includes 5 minute warm-up/cool-down |
|---|---|---|---|---|---|
| **Conditioning Phase** Repeat for one week, three times | 30 seconds | 2 minutes | 8 times | √ | 30 minutes |
| **Week One** | | | | | |
| Long Run | 45 seconds | 2 minutes | 6 times | √ | 26.5 minutes |
| Homework | 45 seconds | 2 minutes | 5 times | √ | 24 minutes |
| Homework | 45 seconds | 2 minutes | 5 times | | 24 minutes |
| **Week Two** | | | | | |
| Long Run | 1 minute | 90 seconds | 9 times | | 32.5 minutes |
| Homework | 1 minute | 90 seconds | 8 times | | 30 minutes |
| Homework | 1 minute | 90 seconds | 7 times | | 27.5 minutes |
| **Week Three** | | | | | |
| Long Run | 90 seconds | 1 minute | 7 times | | 27.5 minutes |
| Homework | 90 seconds | 1 minute | 6 times | | 25 minutes |
| Homework | 90 seconds | 1 minute | 5 times | | 22.5 minutes |

| Week | Fast Interval Run or Fast Walk | Slow Interval Moderate Walk | Quantity How many times this combo is repeated | Check List Stay on track and check when complete | Total Time Includes 5 minute warm-up/ cool-down |
|---|---|---|---|---|---|
| **Week Four** | | | | | |
| Long Run | 2 minutes | 1 minute | 6 times | | 28 minutes |
| Homework | 2 minutes | 1 minute | 4 times | | 22 minutes |
| Homework | 2 minutes | 1 minute | 4 times | | 22 minutes |
| **Week Five** | | | | | |
| Long Run | 3 minutes | 1 minute | 6 times | | 34 minutes |
| Homework | 3 minutes | 1 minute | 5 times | | 30 minutes |
| Homework | 3 minutes | 1 minute | 4 times | | 26 minutes |
| **Week Six** | | | | | |
| Long Run | 4 minutes | 1 minute | 5 times | | 35 minutes |
| Homework | 4 minutes | 1 minute | 4 times | | 30 minutes |
| Homework | 4 minutes | 1 minute | 4 times | | 30 minutes |
| **Week Seven** | | | | | |
| Long Run | 5 minutes | 1 minute | 5 times | | 40 minutes |
| Homework | 5 minutes | 1 minute | 4 times | | 34 minutes |
| Homework | 5 minutes | 1 minute | 4 times | | 34 minutes |
| **Week Eight** | **Recovery Week** | | | | |
| Long Run | 5 minutes | 1 minute | 5 times | | 40 minutes |
| Homework | 5 minutes | 1 minute | 4 times | | 34 minutes |
| Homework | 5 minutes | 1 minute | 4 times | | 34 minutes |
| **Week Nine** | | | | | |
| Long Run | 6 minutes | 1 minute | 5 times | | 45 minutes |
| Homework | 6 minutes | 1 minute | 4 times | | 38 minutes |
| Homework | 6 minutes | 1 minute | 4 times | | 38 minutes |
| **Week Ten** | | | | | |
| Long Run | 7 minutes | 1 minute | 5 times | | 50 minutes |
| Homework | 7 minutes | 1 minute | 4 times | | 42 minutes |
| Homework | 7 minutes | 1 minute | 4 times | | 42 minutes |

| Week | Fast Interval<br>Run or Fast Walk | Slow Interval<br>Moderate Walk | Quantity<br>How many times this combo is repeated | Check List<br>Stay on track and check when complete | Total Time<br>Includes 5 minute warm-up/cool-down |
|---|---|---|---|---|---|
| **Week Eleven** | | | | | |
| Long Run | 8 minutes | 1 minute | 6 times | | 64 minutes |
| Homework | 8 minutes | 1 minute | 5 times | | 55 minutes |
| Homework | 8 minutes | 1 minute | 5 times | | 55 minutes |
| **Week Twelve** | | **Taper Week** | | | |
| Long Run | 6 minutes | 1 minute | 5 times | | 45 minutes |
| Homework | 4 minutes | 1 minute | 4 times | | 30 minutes |
| **Race/Goal Day** | | **Congratulations!** | | | |
| At your comfort level, aim for: | 5–8 minute intervals | 1 minute | 5K distance | | Record your time! |

CONGRATULATIONS; EMBARKING ON a 5K program takes courage! Once I completed my first 5K I built on that experience and went on to do more. I started to increase my distances over time, making sure that I used trusted training programs that were very gradual and injury-prevention focused. Keep traveling your road to limitless and showing up for the game. By doing so you are sending the world a clear message that everyone can be an athlete.

# Big Fit Girl Stretching Routine

A LIMBER BODY is a happy body. From my own experience, I know this to be true and make a full stretching routine a priority after every workout. Stretching isn't just about cooling down and calming your body—it's about the overall health and functionality of your body's biomechanics.

Here are some points to consider:

- Stretching your muscles helps you perform better physically because a body with sound flexibility moves with an optimal range of motion.
- Stretching helps your joints move better because the surrounding muscles are limber, and as a result, move with ease. This can prevent injury.
- Stiff and tight muscles can put stress on the skeleton. This moves your body out of alignment, restricting your movement; in extreme cases this can cause muscle strains and tears and joint issues.

I've admitted before that I haven't always practiced what I've preached, but when it comes to stretching, I have learned my lessons the hard way. I don't want you to go that route. I'm not just recommending a full stretching routine as part of your workout regime; I am saying it *must* be done for long-term, injury-free athleticism. It's that important.

Stretching post-workout is always best because your muscles are warm from being worked; they're more pliable and easily lengthened, giving your body the best opportunity for restoring flexibility. After a heavy workout session of contracting, flexing, and tightening muscles, your body will be begging for it! So let's get to it.

Here is the full stretching routine I do myself and with my athletes after every workout.

### HIP FLEXOR STRETCH

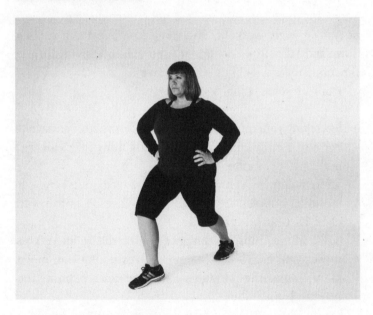

*Target area:* You should feel this stretch in the crease of your hip at the front of your body.

*Execution*: Position your body in a slightly forward lunge position, then push your hips forward while slightly tilting your pelvis up. Hold for thirty seconds, switch sides, and repeat.

*Tip*: Make sure you just tilt your pelvis and not your whole upper body. You're aiming for a very small tilt to the pelvis, nothing dramatic that arches the back.

**HAMSTRING STRETCH**

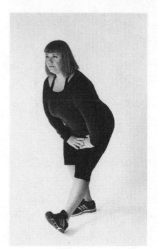
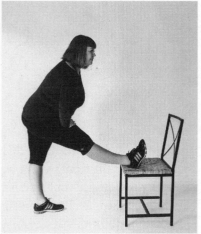

*Target area*: You should feel the hamstring stretch in the upper posterior (back) of your leg between the back of your knee and your bum.

*Execution*: Extend one leg and lean forward, folding the upper body forward from the hips. Your hands can rest gently on your hips or on your upper leg. Hold for thirty seconds, switch sides, and repeat.

*Tip*: Make sure your hands are resting away from your kneecap to avoid adding pressure to the joint while performing this stretch.

## QUADRICEPS STRETCH

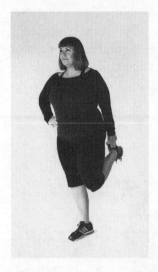 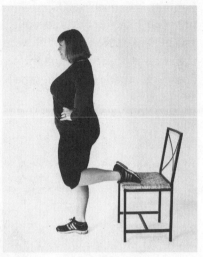

*Target area:* You should feel this stretch between your knee and hip joint in the front of your leg.

*Execution:* Elevate your foot behind you toward your bum. Once your foot is elevated, push your pelvis forward, with your knees together. Hold for thirty seconds, switch sides, and repeat.

*Tip:* This stretch is very important because it targets such a large muscle group; however, many people find it difficult to get into the correct position. If you have difficulty, you can perform a modified version using a chair for assistance.

**CALF STRETCH**

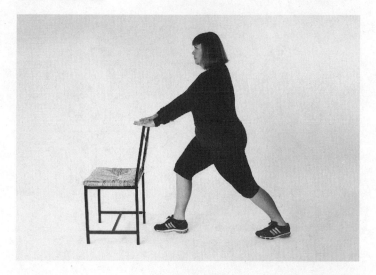

*Target area:* You should feel this stretch in the lower back area of the leg between the ankle and the back of the knee.

*Execution:* Move one leg forward in a slight lunge position and extend the opposing leg straight back, placing your heel flat on the floor. Lean toward a chair (or wall) until you feel the stretch in the calf of the back leg. Hold for thirty seconds, switch sides, and repeat.

*Tip:* Try not to bend your back knee. If you hold your back leg as straight as possible you will enhance the stretch further.

### GLUTEUS MEDIUS STRETCH

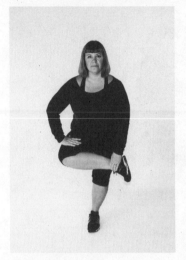 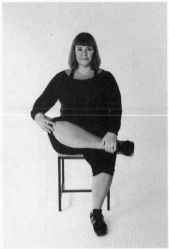

*Target area:* You should feel this stretch from the back of your pelvis into the front of your hip.

*Execution:* Lift up one foot and rest it on the opposing knee, then sit into the stretch, slightly folding your upper body forward. Stretch for thirty seconds, switch sides, and repeat.

*Tips:* If needed, hold onto a chair to stabilize your body, or modify this stretch by sitting in a chair.

## IT BAND STRETCH

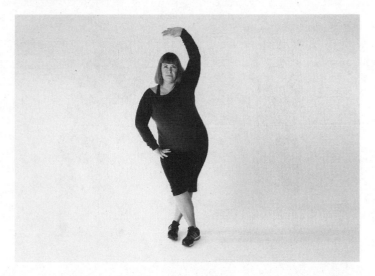

*Target area:* The illiotibial band (or IT band) is a thick piece of connective tissue that runs parallel to the femur bone extending from the hip to the knee. You should feel this stretch down the side of your upper leg.

*Execution:* Cross one foot in front of the other and extend your hip to the side of the front leg. The idea is to push out the IT band with the hip so it can lengthen with the bend. Stretch for thirty seconds, switch sides, and repeat.

*Tip:* By raising your arm overhead (same side as the IT band you are stretching) and leaning to one side, you can lengthen the chain of muscles down the side of your body, which enhances the stretch.

## OBLIQUE AND LAT STRETCH

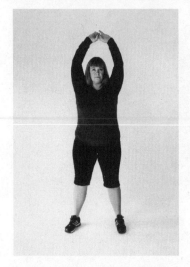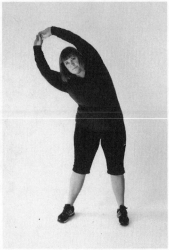

*Target area:* The lats (latissimus dorsi) wrap around your upper rib cage to your back, and your obliques are to the side of your abdominal muscles (abs). You should feel this stretch down the side of your torso.

*Execution:* Raise your arms overhead and lean your body to one side to engage a stretch down the side of your upper body. You will feel the obliques and lats stretch at the same time. Stretch for twenty seconds, switch sides, and repeat.

*Tips:* The further you lean, the deeper the stretch, but do what feels comfortable for you. Keep your upper body square with your feet to execute the stretch the best. Avoid rolling one shoulder forward.

**SHOULDER STRETCH**

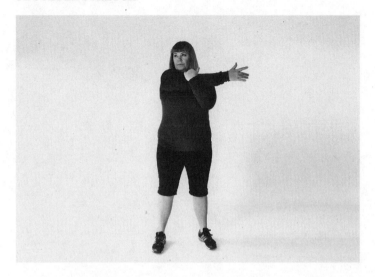

*Target area:* The shoulder is composed of three sections: the rear deltoid, medial deltoid, and anterior deltoid. You should feel this stretch through the shoulders.

*Execution:* Extend one arm across the body and assist the stretch with the other hand to help push the arm across the body. Stretch for twenty seconds, switch sides, and repeat.

*Tips:* While performing this stretch you can create resistance by pushing the assisting hand against the stretching arm. They should be fighting each other. By creating resistance you are engaging the shoulder to stretch further.

**UPPER BACK STRETCH**

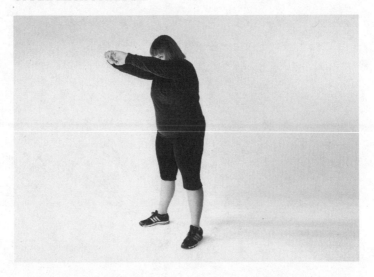

*Target Area:* You should feel this stretch in the upper back from the bottom of your rib cage up to your shoulders.

*Execution:* Reach your arms forward, pressing your chin into your chest, and roll out your upper back like a cat. Stretch for twenty seconds.

*Tips:* Reach as far as you can. You can also extend your hands off to one side, then back to center, then to the other side, stretching different parts of the back.

## CHEST STRETCH

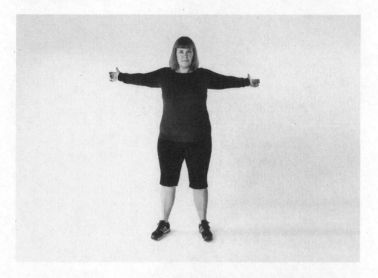

*Target Area:* The chest muscles are also known as the pectoral muscle group (pec minor and major). You should feel this stretch in the chest area across and above the breast.

*Execution:* Standing with your feet slightly apart, extend your arms to the side, then reach your arms back.

*Tip:* You can also perform this stretch with assistance from a doorway. Hold the door frame with your hands, then walk through the door, gently extending the stretch through the chest and into the armpit.

# Safety Rules
## for the Road

WHETHER YOU ARE running, walking, or cycling, being out on the road requires due diligence to remain safe. You can't be certain that drivers will see you when you're crossing the street or cycling on the shoulder of the road—especially when it is dark or it is raining or snowing. Here are my top ten safety recommendations, which I always share with the athletes I train and which are to be followed day or night, rain or shine.

1. Before crossing the street in front of a vehicle, make eye contact with the driver to confirm that he or she has seen you and that it's okay to cross. I also recommend waving your hand or making some other kind of gesture to say thanks and to let the driver know for sure that you are accepting the go-ahead to cross.

2. Avoid wearing headphones. I know, I know—I talk about how music can be motivating while you exercise, and it's an excellent tool to get you through your workouts. But it's never a good idea while you are running, walking, or cycling

outdoors. It's important to be aware of your surroundings at all times and to be able to hear what's behind you and ahead of you. If you must wear headphones, I recommend running or walking at a track, where traffic isn't an issue.

3. Exercise in groups of two or more, especially after dusk. I hate to say this, but the reality is that a woman exercising in the dark by herself is vulnerable. If you must head out alone, stick to busy, well-lit areas where help is only a few steps away.

4. Let people know where you are going. I always give my husband a heads-up about where I am going and how long I am likely to be gone so that if I twist an ankle, get a flat tire, or something else delays me he will have some idea where to find me.

5. Avoid dark clothing and wear reflective clothing or gear when it is dark or raining, since it can be difficult for drivers to see you under such conditions. You can buy reflective vests, jackets with reflective strips, reflective headlamps, or flashing lights to make sure you are seen and safe. This is probably the most important safety recommendation I can make.

6. Choose your routes wisely. If you are heading out on a bike ride, map one out that has either a bike lane or a decent shoulder to ride on. Same with running or walking routes; planning a safe route in advance will ensure that you're not vulnerable to traffic.

7. When you are running, pass others on the sidewalk. I've been in many running groups where the pack is large and faster runners naturally want to pass those who are slower. I've seen some very close calls when a runner steps off the sidewalk to pass on the road. Pass on the sidewalk by saying "On your left" or "Passing from behind." Cyclists typically ride on the road, and single file is always best. But if you

must pass, use your bell to alert the cyclist in front and then say, "Passing on your left." (Never pass on the right.)

8. Take a cell phone so that you can call someone if you get into trouble. I often put my cell phone in my pocket in a Ziploc bag to protect it from sweat.

9. Beware of dogs. I love dogs but they can be dangerous if you are cycling or running. Some canines react to people going fast, and I've seen my cycling partner get nipped at the ankles while we were riding. I also have a client who toppled off her bike and suffered a shoulder injury because an excited dog ran in front of her. Always slow down around dogs, keep a close eye on which direction the leash is going, and maintain eye contact with them to gauge their next move.

10. Run, walk, or cycle in the proper direction, according to the rules of the road. If you are cycling, travel in the same direction as the traffic, meaning your back should be to the cars. If you are walking or running, travel facing the traffic so that you can see what's coming at you. Cyclists are considered traffic, but runners and walkers are considered pedestrians.

# APPENDIX D

## Injury Prevention

IT'S MY GOAL for you to read this book and pursue your athletic dreams safely, healthfully, and realistically. Along the way there will be peaks, valleys, and plateaus in your athletic journey, but injury doesn't have to be a part of your athletic story. I'm happy to say that over many years I've been able to train consistently without any major pushback from my body. As a result, I don't equate exercise with pain, which helps me win part of the mental battle right away. I credit my injury-free history to a number of factors, and I'll share them with you because they are an integral part of smart athleticism. I strongly urge you to follow these tips because injury can kibosh a good training plan in a second, making it difficult for you make a strong comeback.

1. Make sure you have been fitted for athletic shoes for your foot type and that the ones you own are in good shape. I know we've talked about this previously, but it's by no mistake this tip is listed as number one on my injury prevention list. Your shoes should have a good, visible tread on them;

if the tread is worn, then the cushioning is likely worn too. I can tell almost immediately when I need new shoes—new pains start to appear in my body and then it clicks, I need new shoes! A typical estimate for shoe wear is 500K or 6–8 months, depending on use and frequency.

2. Get rid of the mentality of "no pain, no gain." This is an old-school mindset and doesn't apply anymore (at least not in my book). There's a difference between the sensation of burning muscles that are being worked hard and producing lactic acid and that of torn muscles, damaged knee joints, or any extreme discomfort while exercising. No one should try to push you through pain—I don't care who they are! Working through bad pain will likely lead to injury. Exercise can often bring discomfort but you shouldn't experience extreme pain. To prevent injury, it's important to listen to your body's cues and understand what muscle fatigue discomfort feels like compared to pain that could be causing damage. If you feel pain and think damage may be occurring, stop or slow down. Disregard what others might think, or what others might want you to do, and keep your body safe and healthy.

3. Always perform an adequate warm-up. You want to give your brain time to understand what your body is doing, allowing the two to get into a groove with one another. Throwing your body into intense exercise without a proper warm-up sends the mind into fight-or-flight mode and can be exhausting for both the mind and body. A warm-up also gives muscles a chance to become pliable and the synovial fluid in our knee joints time to start responding as a lubricant. Warming up properly can prevent muscle and joint damage; going out cold is taking a risk.

4. Build your fitness routines gradually. You want to avoid crazy intensity. Don't start a fitness program by working

out six days a week—it's too much, too fast for the body to adapt to and will likely result in injury. Gradually build with two days a week of fitness, then after some time, three days, and so on. The key is to listen to your body.

5. Keep your body limber by moving regularly. On the days you're not working out it's okay to keep moving. Go for a walk or a light cycle. If you've been sitting all day at your desk, get up move around and do some stretches. Our bodies are built to move, and when they are sedentary, the body tends to constrict. In a constricted state, muscles shorten, compress, and tighten, and over time become more prone to injury.

6. Stretch at the end of your workouts. Despite leading stretches all the time in my groups, I can be guilty of blowing by my own post-workout stretch, but I do pay for it when I do! Stretching lengthens the muscles after they've been contracting during your exercise, so if you never stretch they just keep forming in that contractive state and become tighter and tighter. Tight muscles can cause limitations in your range of motion and will inevitably compromise your biomechanics, causing injury.

   There are five components to fitness: cardiorespiratory endurance, muscular strength, muscular endurance, body composition, and flexibility. Many of us forget about flexibility, and it's equally important as the other four components, especially when it comes to avoiding injury.

   See page 191 for a full stretching routine to keep your body limber and flexible.

7. Cross-training is another important part of keeping your body strong and staying injury-free. Performing weight-bearing exercise is a great way to cross-train for runners, swimmers, cyclists, dancers, and more. Weight-bearing exercises performed with body weight,

resistance, or free weights build your muscles and keep them strong for all the activities you want to do. If you don't maintain your muscles, you can injure yourself while running or cycling simply because you may not have the strength to perform the given activity.

THESE TIPS ARE a part of smart fitness and by following them, you are taking precautions to keep yourself safe and healthy for the long haul. There are circumstances, however, where you can do everything right and an injury can still occur. Sometimes we can't explain why an injury may happen and it's unfortunate. If an injury is starting to creep into your body, it's always good to be armed with the knowledge of what it is and what it might feel like. Here are some common injuries athletes endure and ways you can deal with them quickly before they become unmanageable.

### Plantar fasciitis

This condition results in pain in the heel and bottom of the foot. It is most extreme with the first steps of the day or when getting up after a period of rest. While the exact cause of plantar fasciitis is unconfirmed, it is thought to be a result of overuse, or an increase in exercise—perhaps too much, too soon—and long periods of standing. It's my humble opinion that poor footwear makes plantar fasciitis worse; I know this from personal experience and talking it out with many clients over the years.

Symptoms: Soreness in the bottom fascia of the foot, sensitivity in the heel.

Treatment: Rest the foot, ice the foot, check your shoes, reduce your fitness routine until it subsides, roll a frozen water bottle under your foot, and seek medical help from a physiotherapist or podiatrist.

### IT band syndrome

Iliotibial band syndrome is one of the most common overuse injuries among runners. It occurs when the iliotibial band, the ligament that runs down the outside of the thigh from the hip to the shin, is tight or inflamed. The IT band attaches to the knee and helps stabilize and move the joint.

Symptoms: You may feel like the side of your knee is burning. When the IT band is extremely tight you may feel the band down the side of your leg, twanging back and forth. The place where it meets your hip may feel sore or burn, or your body may feel like it's out of alignment.

Treatment: Reduce the exercise that is overusing the IT band, stretch out the IT band three to four times a day (see stretching segment, p. 197), and use a foam or rubber roller to roll out your IT band. There are many videos on YouTube that can teach you how to do this—search "IT band + foam roller." If your symptoms don't lessen, seek medical attention through a massage therapist or physiotherapist.

### Shin splints

Shin splints, also known as medial tibial stress syndrome, is almost always related to doing too much, too soon. The body's lack of conditioning gradually causes stress on the tibial bone in the front of the lower leg, earning this condition the catch-all name shin splints.

Symptoms: Soreness in the shin area when walking or running.

Treatment: Back off from your exercise routine; either reduce it or eliminate it for a few days. Ice your shins and check your shoes, and if the condition is extreme or persistent seek medical attention from a physician or physiotherapist.

### Sprained ankle

An ankle sprain can happen when you roll your foot due to walking or running on uneven surfaces, body fatigue, poor footwear, or stepping down off a step or curb. Ankle weakness can also contribute.

Symptoms: Swelling, black and blue bruising, and pain in the ankle.

Treatment: Unfortunately there's not much you can do to prevent this injury, since it has a sudden onset. Now you just need to focus on healing. Have you heard of RICE? It stands for rest, ice, compression, and elevation; all of the above apply for a sprained ankle. The compression can come in the form of a tensor bandage, and with a sprain it's imperative to keep off it as much as possible. After a sprain, you're vulnerable to a reoccurring sprain, so wearing the bandage for stability may help prevent that, along with sound footwear and careful attention to the surface you're walking on.

### Tendonitis (elbow, wrist)

Tendons are tough bands that connect your muscles to your bones and can become inflamed and irritated when certain muscles are overused. Wrist and elbow tendonitis is common when our arms are overused in certain exercises. Some examples are tennis, swimming, or lifting heavy weights too often.

Symptoms: Tenderness, heat in affected area, aching.

Treatment: As with most of these injuries, back off from the exercise that is causing the area grief. The body needs time to reduce inflammation and restore the tendon to a healthy working condition. You can also apply ice for fifteen-minute allotments several times a day to reduce inflammation.

### Achilles tendonitis

Achilles tendonitis is often an overuse injury. It occurs in the Achilles tendon, the band of tissue that connects your calf muscle to your heel bone. This injury has also been attributed to putting too much demand on the body—too much, too soon.

Symptoms: Burning, chronic tightness or soreness right above the back of your heel.

Treatment: Rest, ice, seek physiotherapy.

I've had some issues with my Achilles tendon. I reduced running, iced it, and strengthened my calf muscles by doing calf raises. Achilles tendonitis can be a really nagging injury and you want to be very careful with it, as the Achilles can be difficult to repair. In my case I sought physiotherapy and was fairly quickly back in the game.

### Knee joint pain

Knee joint pain can be very uncomfortable. Even though there may not be a specific injury to the knee joint, pain can occur if you are new to exercise, doing too much too soon, or if the exercise is too high-impact or the surface you are exercising on is too hard. You also may need to take a look at your shoes.

Symptoms: Some knee complications can be more serious, like arthritis, injuries like a meniscus tear, or anterior cruciate ligament (ACL) injury. In these cases your pain will be acute, persistent, and chronic and won't back off with icing or a day or two of rest.

Treatment: General knee pain that isn't acute or chronic can likely be remedied with rest and ice and a survey of your shoes to make sure they are in good working order. If you have any pain that is acute and chronic you should see a medical professional immediately.

ALTHOUGH I AM not a medical professional, I've coached over a thousand athletes of all shapes and sizes, many of whom are exercising for the first time in many years. I've talked through injuries, researched remedies, and gathered advice from appropriate medical professionals to make my training grounds a safe and healthy place for the women I serve. If you take the precautions I've listed you'll have a better chance of avoiding injury, and if you start to feel any of the symptoms described you are now armed with methods to prevent them from escalating. Your health is in your hands and as an athlete it's up to you to listen to and heed your body's warnings so you can stay in the game for the long term.

# THE BIG FIT GLOSSARY

**5K**  The shortest of the common running or walking events covering 5K (3.1 miles).

**10K**  Running or walking event covering 10K (6.2 miles).

**70.3**  Half the distance covered in an Ironman. A total of 113K (70.3 miles), including a 1.9K (1.2-mile) swim, 90K (56-mile) bike ride, and a 21.1K (13.1-mile) run.

**Aerobic**  Activities such as running, swimming, and dancing that require your heart to pump oxygenated blood to the muscles involved in the activity. Benefits include improved cardiovascular efficiency and breathing.

**AMRAP**  "As many reps as possible." Performing a certain number of circuit exercises within a fixed amount of time and repeating as many times as possible.

**Anaerobic**  Activity in which the demand for oxygen exceeds the available oxygen supply. It involves brief high-intensity exercises that rely on sources of energy that are stored in the muscles.

**Athena Division**  A division in triathlon that is for female athletes 165 lbs. and up.

**Athletic stance**  Correct standing position to decrease the risk of injury and to increase power, speed, and strength. Correct stance depends on the sport but in general, it involves: head straight, slight bend in the knees, shoulders back, chest out, and even weight distribution in the feet.

**BMI** "Body Mass Index"; weight (in kg) divided by height (in m²).

**BOSU** An acronym for "Both Sides Up"; a piece of fitness equipment with a flat rigid surface attached to an inflated rubber half ball that is mostly used for balance training.

**Brick** Component of triathlon training encompassing either the swim-bike or bike-run transition. The two workouts are done back to back to replicate the quick transitions that will occur during the race. This is helpful in training muscles for the change between the different disciplines.

**Circuit training** Workout aimed at building muscle endurance and strength involving a quick transition between different stations. Each station will work different muscle groups and requires a certain amount of time or number of reps.

**Clean and jerk** A weightlifting technique that comprises two movements; during the clean, the weightlifter moves the weight from the floor to a position across the chest, and during the jerk, the weightlifter raises the weight above the head.

**Cool-down** Easier exercises that bring the heart rate down and allow the body to return to a resting or near resting state. May include a light jog, walk, or stretches.

**Core** A collection of over fifteen muscles in your pelvis, abdomen, hips, and lower back that when strengthened will assist with balance and stability.

**Cross** The power punch of boxing, where the rear hand throws a straight and powerful punch from the chin, crossing the body and toward the opponent.

**Cross-training** Training in two or more sports or exercises to improve health, efficiency, and development of various muscles.

**DOMS** "Delayed onset muscle soreness." Muscle fatigue, weakness, pain, and stiffness that usually presents itself hours to days after exercise.

**Duathlon** Event or race involving a running leg followed by a biking leg and then a second running leg.

**Electrolytes** Chemicals in the body such as sodium, calcium, and potassium that carry an electrical charge that helps the body function. Electrolyte replacements during strenuous activities are important to maintain muscle contractions and normal functioning.

**Endorphins** Chemicals released by the body as a response to pain or physical exertion that allow humans to endure strenuous activity by interacting with receptors in the brain to minimize the perception of pain. They trigger a positive feeling in the body and are responsible for the "runner's high."

**Endurance** The ability to sustain exercise or activity for an extended period of time without fatigue.

**Fartlek** Means "speed play" in Swedish and includes varying the speed and terrain during long distance runs.

**Fighting stance** Position used in boxing in which your body is slightly turned with your non-dominant foot forward, knees slightly bent, and hands up at eye level without blocking your eyes.

**Flexibility** The quality of having a wide range of motion in your joints and muscles, allowing them to move freely.

**Foam roller** A tube covered with foam that can be used for stretching and flexibility.

**Free weights** Used for weightlifting; weights such as kettle bells and dumbbells that are not attached to another piece of equipment. These will help improve overall strength and power as you use stabilizing muscles to lift.

**Freestyle**  The most common stroke used in competitive swimming, involving swimming on your stomach with alternating strokes with your arms while maintaining a constant kick.

**Fueling**  Eating and drinking appropriately prior to or during strenuous activity to improve intensity and results of the workout.

**Gait**  How an individual walks or runs.

**Gels**  Supplemental energy gels that are used to replenish the body's carbohydrate stores that are depleted during activity.

**HAES**  "Health at Every Size" is a movement that supports people in adopting healthy habits for the sake of health and well-being, rather than weight control.

**Half-marathon**  Running event that covers a 21.1K (13.1-mile) course.

**Hatha yoga**  Gentle, slow-paced, and simple yoga with little flow between poses. Includes stretching and basic breathing exercises.

**High impact**  Fast and high-intensity exercises that increase the amount of strain and force placed on the body.

**HIIT**  "High intensity interval training"; involves quick bursts of exercises followed by short recovery periods that aim to increase heart rate, improve the cardiovascular system, and increase both aerobic and anaerobic metabolism.

**Hill repeats**  Running up and down the same hill to help build strength, efficiency, and speed.

**Hook**  A short sideways punch delivered to a boxing opponent's head with the fist horizontal and elbow bent.

**Hot yoga**  A style of yoga done in humid and hot conditions in order to increase flexibility.

**Intensity**  The amount of power the body uses during exercises.

**Interval training**  Alternating periods of low-intensity activity with periods of high-intensity activity in between rest periods to help increase fitness and burn more calories.

**Ironman** Long distance triathlon event consisting of a 3.9K (2.4-mile) swim, 180.25K (112-mile) cycle, and a 42.2K (26.2-mile) run.

**Jab** A fast and quick boxing punch with the leading hand moving straight from the chin to the opponent.

**Lactic acid** A metabolic by-product produced by muscles when they are deprived of oxygen during activity. Buildup can cause muscle fatigue, cramping, and pain.

**Low impact** Easier and lighter exercises with lower intensity to decrease the amount of strain and force placed on the body.

**Metabolism** The chemical and physical processes that occur in the body in order to maintain the energy required for proper functioning.

**Olympic bar** Used for exercise and weightlifting, a long bar that can hold weights at either end to increase or decrease the weight of the bar.

**Olympic triathlon** A triathlon course consisting of a 1,500m swim, 40K (24.9-mile) bike ride, and 10K (6.2-mile) run.

**On-your-left** What you yell as a courtesy while biking when you want to pass someone on their left side.

**Passive recovery** Exercising at a low intensity on purpose, to help your body recover from high-intensity exercises.

**Periodization** Periodization is a style of training where the training plan is broken into different periods. Each period serves a purpose in reaching an end goal. An example is athletic training stages: conditioning, endurance, power, and maintenance stages.

**Personal best** Also know as PB. One's best time or score in their event.

**Plank** Exercise using core strength that involves maintaining an iso-metric position that resembles a push-up (on elbows and toes) for the longest time possible. Weight should be distributed on the elbows, forearms, and toes with your back completely flat and body in a straight line.

**Power yoga** A faster moving form of yoga that helps increase stamina, flexibility, and strength, and builds internal heat.

**Pyramids** Fitness training method in which you start with a lower number of reps and increase repetitions for each set, and then reverse the process and go from the higher to lower reps.

**Quadriceps** The group of four muscles at the front of the leg above the knee.

**Recovery** The time it takes you to recover or catch your breath and regain normal breathing.

**Rep** Short for "repetition." The number of times you can perform a specific exercise.

**Resistance training** Exercises using equipment that applies resistance in order to increase muscle tone, strength, mass, and endurance.

**Resting heart rate** Heart rate when not doing any physical activity.

**Restorative yoga** Form of yoga aimed at providing emotional, mental, and physical relaxation.

**RICE** "Rest, ice, compression, elevation." A method used to help treat injuries.

**Roundhouse** A circular kick used in kickboxing.

**Shavasana** Yoga pose aimed at fully relaxing the mind and body, performed by lying on your back with arms and legs spread out.

**Set** The number of cycles of reps that you can complete.

**Shin splints** Pain along the tibia (shin bone) caused by overuse of muscles, stress fractures, over-pronation of the feet, or weakness in the stabilizing muscles of the hips or core.

**Southpaw** The stance of a lefthanded fighter who jabs with the right hand and throws power punches with the left hand.

**Split stance** Standing position with one foot a few feet in front of the other that improves balance and strength to the core and lower body.

**Sprint triathlon** The shortest triathlon distance consisting of a 750m swim, 20K (12.4-mile) bike ride, and a 5K (3.1-mile) run.

**Stability ball** A large exercise ball used for stretching, core exercises, balance, and strength training.

**Streamline** A drill used in swimming to help improve comfort, efficiency, and speed.

**Strength training** Fitness method to help build endurance, strength, and muscle size using resistance and weights.

**Superset** Performing multiple exercises in a row with minimal rest in between to help improve the cardiovascular system.

**Tabata** High-intensity interval training usually consisting of twenty seconds of high-intensity training with ten seconds of rest.

**Talk test** An easy way to measure intensity during exercise. You should be able to talk while performing moderate-intensity exercises. While doing high-intensity exercises, you will be unable to say more than a few words without pausing for a breath.

**Target heart rate** Specific to a person's gender, age, or physical fitness, the minimum number of heartbeats in a specific time period to ensure optimal cardiovascular fitness.

**Tempo** The rhythm you move in during exercise.

**Transition** Moving from one exercise to another.

**Triathlon** An athletic event involving three events: swimming, cycling, and running.

**Trigger point** Formed by stressed or injured muscles, an area with musculoskeletal tightness and pain.

**TRX** A suspension training technique that simultaneously helps develop balance, strength, core stability, and flexibility.

**Unilateral training** Training one side of the body at a time.

**Uppercut**  In boxing, an upward punch aiming at the opponent's jaw.

**V-Sit**  A specific sitting position that is effective in building core strength by working multiple core areas at the same time.

**Warm up**  Stretching or loosening the muscles in preparation for exercise.

**Wicking material**  Fabric that draws moisture such as sweat away from the body.

**WOD**  Common CrossFit term that stands for "workout of the day."

**Yin yoga**  A slow-paced yoga style that targets connective tissue with poses that are held for longer periods of time.

# NOTES

## Introduction

1. "100 Million Dieters, $20 Billion: The Weight-Loss Industry by the Numbers," ABC *News*, May 8, 2012, http://abcnews.go.com/ Health/100-million-dieters-20-billion-weight-loss-industry/ story?id=16297197.

## Chapter One

1. Kelsey Miller, "We Let You Down and We're Going to Fix It," Refinery 29, September 26, 2016, http://www.refinery29.com/ 2016/09/123687/plus-size-american-women-67-percent-essay.

## Chapter Two

1. Michelle Paccagnella, "Using mental rehearsal to prepare for officiating," Australian Sports Commission, http://www.ausport. gov.au/sportsofficialmag/mental_preparation/using_mental_ rehearsal_to_prepare_for_officiating.

## Chapter Four

1. Melissa Lem, "How Wearing the Wrong Bra Can Be Bad for Your Health," *The Steven and Chris Show,* July 13, 2015, http://www.cbc. ca/stevenandchris/health/abcs-of-bra-health.

**Chapter Six**

1.  "Sodium: How to tame your salt habit," Mayo Clinic, April 16, 2016, http://www.mayoclinic.org/healthy-lifestyle/nutrition-and-healthy-eating/in-depth/sodium/art-20045479.
2.  "Dietary Sodium, Heart Disease and Stroke," Heart and Stroke Foundation, http://www.heartandstroke.com/site/c.ikIQLcMWJtE/b.5263133/k.696/Dietary_sodium_heart_disease_and_stroke.htm.
3.  Sandi Busch, "USDA Protein Requirements in Grams," SF Gate, http://healthyeating.sfgate.com/usda-protein-requirements-grams-8619.html.

**Chapter Seven**

1.  James McIntosh, "Does the menstrual cycle affect sporting performance?," *Medical News Today*, July 22, 2015, http://www.medicalnewstoday.com/articles/297154.php.
2.  A. Campbell and H. Hausenblas, "Effects of Exercise Interventions on Body Image," *Journal of Health Psychology* 14, no. 6 (2009): 780-93.
3.  N. Zhu, "Cardiorespiratory fitness and cognitive function in middle age: the CARDIA study," *Neurology*, April 2, 2015, https://www.ncbi.nlm.nih.gov/pubmed/24696506.

# INDEX